W9-CTN-378

FORBIDDEN CURES

Proven natural treatments the medical establishment won't let you have

By Dr. Benjamin Ross

Whistleblowers, Truth-Tellers and Vigilant Defenders of Your Right to Know!

Here are just some of the 19 great doctors, researchers and health practitioners on...

The Health Sciences Institute Advisory Panel

Martin Milner, N.D., is Professor of Cardiovascular and Pulmonary Medicine, National College of Naturopathic Medicine and Bastyr University. He also serves as President and Medical Director of the Center for Natural Medicine.

Randall Wilkinson, M.D., left private practice to dedicate all of his time to research. A specialist in environmental medicine, he brought our members the tocotrienols breakthrough for fighting heart disease and cancer. He is currently conducting anti-aging research.

Elson M. Haas, M.D., integrates traditional Chinese therapies with natural healing methods from the West. His books include *The Detox Diet* and the classic *Staying Healthy with Nutrition*, used in many alternative health schools. He serves as Medical and Creative Director at the Preventive Medical Center of Marin.

Ann Louise Gittleman, Ph.D., C.N.S. As millions of television viewers have seen on "Dr. Phil" and "The View," she's constantly breaking new ground in all aspects of health from natural hormone replacement to effective and safe weight loss. Dr. Gittleman is the award-winning author of 20 books on health and healing, with more than 3.5 million copies in print.

Kohhei (Tadahiro) Makise, M.D., Medical Director of the Kyoto Imadagawo Makise Clinic, Kyoto. Considered one of the most cutting-edge physicians in Japan, Dr. Makise recently scored a breakthrough in treating severe dermatitis without cortisone.

Allan Spreen, M.D. has helped spread the truth about natural medicine and expose common medical myths through his book *Nutritionally Incorrect – Why the American Diet is Dangerous & How to Defend Yourself*. He's known as the "Nutrition Physician."

Claus Martin, M.D., is Medical Director of the Four Seasons Medical Center and Clinic, Rottach-Egern, Germany. He's a leading expert in therapies to retard the aging process and regenerate organs with a natural form of genetic engineering.

Hyla Cass, M.D., serves as Assistant Clinical Professor of Psychiatry at the UCLA School of Medicine and is a distinguished spokesperson, consultant and educator in complementary medicine and psychiatry. She specializes in alternative solutions to psychiatric disorders, with the aim of replacing prescription medications with alternatives. Dr. Cass is the author of seven books including *All About Herbs*.

Eric Berg, D.C. is a renowned nutritional researcher, chiropractor and founder of the Health and Wellness Center in Alexandria, Virginia who certifies M.D.'s and D.C.'s in his techniques. He originated the Body Restoration Technique, invented the Acoustic Heart Monitor, and is a past associate professor at Howard University. His latest book, *Dr. Berg's Body Shape Diets*, shares his discoveries about the hormone-body distortion connection.

Jon Barron is one of the world's leading researchers and educators in the fields of nutrition and herbal therapy. His book, *Lessons from the Miracle Doctors: Step-by-Step Guide to Optimum Health and Relief from Catastrophic Illness*, is widely hailed as a classic in the field of alternative medicine.

Table of Contents

Table of Contents

Can you believe it? Read on to learn more...

Chapter One

They won't let us have the cures!

Imagine if someone you loved died of cancer, and you found out there was a cure that no one told you about.

If you underwent a heart bypass, would it bother you to learn you didn't have to? That a cheap herb solves most heart problems, and does it for pennies—but no one told you?

If you've been on insulin for years, would you get angry if you discovered other people have cleared up diabetes within weeks, without drugs?

Suppose you had to rush your asthmatic child to an emergency room several times a year. What would you say if you learned there was a cure all along—and nobody told you?

Would that make you angry?

Then get ready to get angry. Because...

Cures *do* exist for cancer, heart disease, diabetes, asthma, allergies, pain, cataracts, osteoporosis, arthritis, fatigue, Alzheimer's and more. And you'll learn about them right in this book. But our medical establishment does *everything in its power to keep them away from you.*

And don't blame your doctor! You see, this powerful multi-billion-dollar industry controls all medical information. They effectively shut down all dissent. Step out of line and you lose your right to practice.

I know, because it happened to me!

They took away my license and livelihood just for using treatments they don't like. Now I've got nothing to lose, so I'm going to blow the lid off their scam.

In this book, you'll discover treatments <u>no one else will tell you about</u>, not even alternative doctors, because they fear what might happen to them.

Doctors aren't free to tell you the truth

I'm not the only doctor they've victimized. Dozens of alternative doctors have been through the same thing, not to mention supplement makers, and even health information publishers.

<u>In the state of Washington, the "health police" are investigating and harassing one out of every three alternative M.D.'s in the state</u>.

They've taken away one doctor's license and totally put him out of business.

It's a wonder there are any alternative doctors left free to practice

Just listen to Dr. W's story. He knows all about the brutal attacks and intimidation.

With guns drawn, FDA goons busted down the doors of his office and proceeded to haul away patient records, supplements, medicines and office equipment. It was two weeks before he could reopen his clinic and start seeing patients again.

And that was just the beginning of a two-and-a-half-year nightmare that cost Dr. W and his family $350,000. He was hauled before two grand juries and, at one point, he had eleven attorneys defending his case.

Other alternative doctors advised him to do what they did: Give up and knuckle under to the authorities. Instead, Dr. W fought back—and won. But he's the exception.

His "crime"? Prescribing preservative-free vitamins

No charges were ever brought against Dr. W. And what was this all about? Why, the FDA had gone through his dumpster and found bottles of vitamin B-12 they said were contaminated. Well, they *were* in a dumpster. They *might* have been contaminated!

Of course, this case was really about the FDA trying to intimidate a leading alternative doctor, a man who served on the faculty of an alternative medicine university and—gasp!—wrote books. (The FDA has literally burned books that contained information they don't approve of.)

As a practicing D.O., an osteopath, I was on probation for ten years while the government-appointed "health police" second-guessed every single thing I did. For ten years, they looked for an excuse to put me out of business.

I stopped an asthma attack with the touch of my hands, and lost my license as a result!

Establishment medicine is enraged by people like Dr.

W and me who help patients get well the natural way, without drugs and surgery. <u>They do everything they can to shut us up and shut us down</u>.

If you think it's far-fetched to say that cures actually exist, and that people like me are persecuted for using them, let me set you straight.

One of the things they nailed me for during my ten years on probation was the time I treated a boy who was suffering from an asthma attack.

This boy's mother took him to an emergency room because she was afraid he was going to die. The boy was one of my patients, and had been since he was a baby. But his mom was so frightened by this attack she didn't come to me, she went straight to the ER.

What happened there was worse than anything she could imagine. The attending physician in the ER overdosed the child and the seizure got worse. The mother saw that what they were doing in the ER might kill her boy, so she picked him up and left. She came straight to my office.

I performed osteopathic manipulations on the kid and the seizure stopped. Problem over.

The Board of Physicians in my state investigated the incident and claimed I'd done the wrong thing. The boy should have gone to the ER, they said. I explained that the boy had *come* from the ER. The ER *caused the problem*.

The Board didn't care. The kid belonged in the ER. I

fixed the problem the ER caused, just by performing manipulations with my hands. They didn't care.

The boy got well. The mother wasn't complaining. They didn't care.

Multiply that incident by ten years of crazy accusations just like it. That's what I went through. It destroyed my career and it nearly destroyed my life.

I'm a married man with eight kids to support. Yes, you heard right. Eight kids.

Yet I was thrown out of work by our insane medical establishment. I'm now in a new career, doing research, and I love it. My attitude is the Good Lord wanted me to be doing something else. But...

What the medical establishment did is very wrong

That's why I decided to send this book to you. It's about time somebody blew the whistle. You have no idea how many exciting treatments are kept away from you.

I'm angry not just because of what establishment medicine did to me, but because of what they're doing to *you and your loved ones*—to all of us.

All I had to do was find a new career. But I believe there are people out there suffering—or even dead—because they never learned about the treatments you'll read about in this little book. That little boy with asthma might well be dead. Thank God, I still had my license to practice then, but what about next time?

13

I'm writing you on behalf of a group that's working to right these wrongs

That group is called Health Sciences Institute. They've been around for eleven years now. Eleven glorious years of bringing Americans blacklisted, banned and forbidden health solutions from all over the world.

HSI doesn't depend on one medical guru. We have an Advisory Panel with no less than 19 distinguished doctors, researchers and scientists who are dedicated to a simple idea:

Somewhere on this lovely blue planet, if you just look hard enough...

You can find a cure for just about <u>every</u> disease

Keep reading and you'll learn about quite a few of the cures in this book. You'll see the proof, including the kind of scientific studies that supposedly don't exist for natural therapies—if you believe the "health police."

What's more, Health Sciences Institute doesn't manufacture or sell these amazing health solutions. They don't profit in any way. Their only mission is to tell you the truth.

You'll read real-life stories from people who got the help they needed. Wouldn't you want to know about:

- **Cancer patients who got totally well**—including the worst case of leukemia the Mayo Clinic had seen in 20 years? (See Chapters 2, 3 and 12)

- A woman who was able to **get off insulin in only six weeks**—after nine years on drugs? (See Chapter 4)

- **A real answer to arthritis.** Not just a painkiller —a *real solution*, with a success rate of almost 100%?!

- **Nutrients that stop Alzheimer's and reverse it!** They work for everyday "forgetfulness," too. <u>You could reverse 12 years of memory loss</u>! (Chapter 6)

- One Asian herb that **solves nearly every heart problem**. Could there be a natural superstar that cuts bad cholesterol and cures angina better than the best prescription drugs? See for yourself in Chapter 5.

- **The "missing link" in your body's system for making energy.** This could be the real reason you're tired all the time. Now for the first time you can get this rare nutrient in supplement form. (Chapter 11)

- Natural eye drops that **beat cataracts**? Success rate: close to 100 percent. *Everybody* in the test got better. (Chapter 9)

- A new herb you've never heard of that <u>wipes out prostate tumors</u> AND shrinks enlarged prostates? So valuable that the country that grows it doesn't want to sell it! (See Chapter 8)

They can't silence 90,000 of us!

This book is a free gift to you from Health Sciences Institute, alternative medicine's foremost global information network. We're 90,000 dedicated doctors, researchers and health-conscious people like you.

If HSI practiced medicine, the "health police" wouldn't let us reveal the shocking information in this book. Did you know that supplement makers aren't allowed to tell you all the ways their products can benefit your health? It's against the law. But WE can. We are strictly information providers, so we're protected by the First Amendment.

We're free to speak our minds. That's why today's most gifted researchers are constantly telling *us* what they can't tell you. Get ready for some very big surprises.

Then, we hope you'll decide to help support our work by becoming a member. We've prepared some very special gifts and privileges for you, as you'll see in the last chapter.

PLUS: A natural way to control your bladder (good-bye Depends—see Chapter 10) …Too much calcium is not making your bones stronger. It's making you sick! (Chapter 13) …**And more**.

We've got a lot to cover! So let's get started...

Chapter Two

Total remission for more than half of these cancer patients

Thanks to natural food extracts revealed for the first time in our pages...

If you're being treated for cancer, the most wonderful words you can hear are, "You're in TOTAL remission. We can't find any cancer cells in your body."

In a 1995 study, <u>more than half of the cancer patients in this particular study heard those joyful words: TOTAL REMISSION</u>. To be exact...

As many as 66 percent of the participants got as close as you ever get to a complete cure

Listen up, because we're going to tell you about a <u>safe, natural cancer remedy</u> you'd NEVER hear about in America if it weren't for Health Sciences Institute. This natural wonder is an HSI first.

We published the news in 2000, so our readers and their loved ones have reaped the benefit for nearly seven years while most people knew nothing about it.

As often happens, other alternative newsletters picked up the story after we broke it, but not as many as you might expect! The FDA and the rest of the establishment have frightened them away from alternative cancer therapies.

A booster rocket for your immune system

The cancer therapy I'm talking about is a mushroom extract pioneered in Japan and used there for years. The Japanese have known about the healing properties of mushrooms for *centuries*. Now, scientists have stepped in and thoroughly proven the medicinal power of certain mushrooms.

But this new, revolutionary mushroom extract goes far beyond any previous discovery. <u>It's made from a special hybrid of several kinds of mushrooms known to be powerful disease-fighters</u>.

What's more, Japanese scientists have identified the amazing ingredient. It's a biochemical so powerful that dozens of studies *prove* it's one of the world's safest and most potent immune-system stimulators. The mushroom extract nearly...

Triples your immune system's power

It increases a key measure of immune system activity by as much as <u>300 percent</u>! I'm talking about your own "natural killer cells." As the name suggests, these cells can penetrate and kill cancer cells, *but only if your immune system is healthy*.

This is an absolute scientific fact, but it's one that America's "cancer industry" criminally ignores. Instead, they bombard patients with radiation and chemotherapy that actually *destroy* the immune system.

Their approach is, "We'll give you poison, and if you're lucky the poison will kill the cancer before it kills *you*."

A biochemical time bomb

Your natural killer cells decline with age and illness. But when they're healthy they can identify a cancer cell, latch on to its outer membrane, and inject a biochemical "time bomb."

Within five minutes, this natural defense explodes and destroys an enemy cell. Then the natural killer cell can move on and kill another.

A healthy natural killer cell can even kill two cancer cells at a time!

<u>And scientists have demonstrated the mushroom extract boosts natural killer cell activity by as much as 300 percent</u>!

But the new extract goes way beyond that. It increases immune system function in a half dozen different ways. <u>T-cell activity goes up as much as 200 percent</u> and interferon levels increase, too.

In other words, <u>your body can heal itself</u> if given the right tools. The mushroom extract feeds your immune cells what they need, and they do the rest. No wonder American millionaires used to fly in their own private supply from Japan! Now I've got more good news...

You don't have to fly to Japan anymore

You can now obtain this powerful immune-booster legally right here in the United States. Best of all, you'll learn about how you can safely take it to *help your body fight off* disease. And...

It's a food that's totally safe

Let's make one thing crystal clear: This is a totally harmless FOOD. There are NO side effects and <u>it can't hurt you</u>.

Carol from Grand Junction, Colorado, found the extract actually *reduces* the dreaded side effects of chemotherapy. "I didn't have the nausea, the weight loss, or the lack of energy that's usually associated with my chemotherapy treatments."

It's not just you, Carol! Studies show that patients suffer less from chemotherapy and radiation when they supplement with mushroom extract.

This cancer treatment makes you feel <u>better</u> instead of sick and weak

Jacqueline from Tucson exclaims. "The change in energy and strength were dramatic. For the first time in two years my energy is great!"

Jacqueline started taking the mushroom extract AFTER finishing radiation treatment for breast cancer. Now she tells everyone about it, because <u>even healthy people can benefit from this astonishing immune system booster</u>. She adds...

"If it weren't for Health Sciences Institute, I would have never known..."

And what's the cost of this medical miracle? At the recommended dosage it'll cost less than ten bucks a day. Not as cheap as vitamin C, I'll admit, but it's peanuts compared to the cost of medical treatments.

81 percent success rate

Remember the study I told you about earlier, where 54 percent of the patients experienced *total remission*? I left something out. *Out of the 11 patients in the study an additional 27 percent* experienced partial remission. So the mushroom extract helped patients <u>an unbelievable 81 percent of the time</u>.

What's more, a healthy person can take the mushroom extract to *prevent* the spread of the disease—in much smaller doses and at lower cost. When you become a member of Health Sciences Institute, you'll receive all the information you need to decide.

You see, every new member of HSI receives a free Special Research Alert called *6 Natural Cancer Cures THEY DON'T WANT YOU TO HAVE*. The report includes information about the mushroom extract PLUS five other powerful cancer remedies. We don't profit from your decision—we aren't connected in any way to the manufacturer or the sale of any supplement.

We'd have our hands full if we did, because there are effective, proven cancer remedies you never hear about!

How can this be? Why haven't you heard about these cures before? Are doctors—even alternative doctors— holding out on you? Let me explain what's going on...

How the authorities keep natural cures away from you

The "health police" turn up their noses at vitamins and minerals, but they don't mind if you take them. And when it comes to natural cures for headaches or colds, they don't like them, but they figure "no harm done."

But a cure for *cancer*? Watch out! They drop the atom bomb on you. NOTHING brings out the rage and contempt of the medical industry like an alternative therapy aimed at cancer. They'll do anything—ANYTHING— whatever it takes—to discredit alternative cancer treatments and get them banned.

What's more, it's easy to do. <u>No cancer treatment is going to save everybody</u>. So it's easy to focus on the patients who don't make it—and then call the doctor a quack.

Worse yet, most cancer patients don't turn to alternatives till they've tried everything else. After they've waited too long and their conventional doctors tell them nothing more can be done...after their bodies are ravaged by toxic chemotherapy and radiation...guess what? They go to an alternative doctor.

To the "health police" attacking alternative doctors who take on cancer cases is like shooting fish in a barrel.

The authorities LOVE it, and their press releases have the nerve to brag how they've saved you from phony treatments. Their errand boys in the mainstream press dutifully report it all as a "public service."

Don't you believe it.
There are many blacklisted
cancer treatments that <u>work</u>

But the kind of doctors who write alternative health bulletins have to be very careful, especially if they still see patients. They can lose their right to practice.

Health Sciences Institute doesn't have that problem— HSI provides health information. Since we don't practice medicine, we're totally protected by the First Amendment. (Remember that?)

So we've collected the very latest and best alternative cancer treatments into a Special Research Alert called *6 Natural Cancer Cures THEY DON'T WANT YOU TO HAVE*—and we rush a FREE copy to every new member.

Look for your Membership Application in this envelope…

Wonderful as the mushroom remedy is, there are many other banned and forbidden treatments in the next few pages: Read all about the discoveries for fighting diabetes (Chapter 4), heart disease (Chapter 5), Alzheimer's (Chapter 6)—and more!

Keep reading!

Chapter Three

Forbidden cancer treatment—From the same man who discovered vitamin C!

Establishment doctors turned their backs on it

A Hungarian doctor discovered vitamin C and got a Nobel Prize for it in 1937. But here's something very few people know: The same doctor ALSO identified a natural cancer-fighting compound in wheat germ.

Establishment medicine is so hostile to natural therapies, even winning a Nobel Prize doesn't protect you. True, the doctor's findings were published about 40 years ago by the National Academy of Sciences. That's the top of the line when it comes to scientific prestige.

But his startling discovery was ignored by a medical community hell-bent on killing cancer cells with chemo and radiation.

You don't have to pay the price for their tragic greed and ignorance, because alternative doctors found a way to go forward with the research on wheat germ.

The Almighty gets some of the credit

It wasn't easy. At one point, the money situation was so hopeless the doctor was about to cut half of all his research, so he got down on his knees and prayed to the Virgin Mary.

The next day, an investor came through with a check for $100,000. The grateful doctor named the supplement "Avemar," short for Ave Maria, which is Latin for "Hail Mary."

Supplement reduced the effects of cancer by nearly 67 percent

In a study of patients with colorectal cancer, upwards of 67% of patients had improved quality of life, longer life and even complete remission using the supplement.

Wait, it gets even better. In the same study, those on the wheat germ extract slashed their risk of some form of a relapse nearly 80 percent!

Studies have also shown that standard therapies such as chemo are up to *twelve times more effective* when the patients also take the natural immune-system booster discovered by the Hungarian doctor.

What's more, patients who took the wheat germ compound suffered much less from chemotherapy's dreaded side effects. The supplement reduced nausea, fatigue, weight loss, and immune-system suppression. Many patients *got better*, and they *felt better* while they were at it.

This wonder food is not just for cancer

You'll be thrilled to know that <u>healthy people can benefit, too</u>. The supplement is an all-around immune system booster!

Please be aware that you won't reap the benefits just by eating wheat germ from the supermarket. This special supplement is a compound extracted from wheat germ and *fermented* by an exclusive, patented technique. It's probably not a good option if you're allergic to wheat, but other than that, it's...

"...as safe as whole wheat bread"

...according to an independent panel of experts. It's actually classified as a food in Hungary, where it's now a standard cancer therapy. It's also available in—and deemed safe by—many other countries from Switzerland to Australia.

It would take too much space to tell everything you need to know about this wonderful discovery. When you join Health Sciences Institute, we'll rush you a free Special Research Alert called *6 Natural Cancer Cures THEY DON'T WANT YOU TO HAVE*.

In fact, all new members receive EIGHT free Special Research Alerts—a complete library of cures the "health police" would keep from you—if they could.

The wheat germ extract is just one example of the awesome health breakthroughs you never hear about. *Let me tell you about the diabetes discovery...*

Chapter Four

Get off insulin in six weeks?

This woman did it after nine years on prescription drugs

If only she'd known about the "blood sugar supplement" she could have prevented the problem before it started!

June, a 56-year-old woman living in Dubuque with diabetes, had been on insulin and oral prescription medications for 9 years when she agreed to test a new natural solution.

Within six weeks she stopped not only her insulin but another prescription drug as well.

You heard right: In six weeks an alternative doctor solved a problem that mainstream medicine couldn't handle in 9 years and after burning up thousands of dollars. It costs the typical diabetic around $10,000 a year for treatment.

Can you imagine? Conventional medicine soaked this woman for maybe $90,000 to treat a medical problem that plant remedies cured in no time at all!

A standard diabetes test showed the lady went from severely diabetic to healthy in the course of the treatment.

Even healthy folks can benefit from this HSI "first"!

The new diabetes solution is a great example of how

you benefit from being part of the Health Sciences Institute network. Thanks to our inside, confidential sources, we were able to follow the development and testing process and bring this breakthrough to our readers as soon as it was available.

What's more, we were able to secure a members-only discount. But the breakthrough almost didn't happen! Let me explain...

Reluctant researcher didn't want to invent the formula!

This story has a happy ending, but it was a close call. The acclaimed researcher who found this remedy wanted nothing to do with creating a diabetes treatment!

It's true. His name is Jon Barron. We know Jon well because he's a member of our Health Sciences Institute Advisory Panel. He got there by racking up one of the world's most impressive records as a researcher and educator in nutrition and herbal therapy.

For years, Jon turned down the idea that he should come up with a supplement for battling diabetes. He thought it would be a mistake to use herbs and nutrients to manage the *symptoms* of diabetes. The responsible approach is to get at the root cause, mainly the way we eat.

40 percent of us are on our way to diabetes

What changed Jon's mind was the galloping diabetes epidemic all around us. Nearly 20 million Americans already have full-blown diabetes, and up to 40 percent of the rest of us are pre-diabetic.

Jon Barron decided the diabetes epidemic is so severe we can't wait for people to be "good." Half of us will be dead before that happens.

Diabetes is the Number 6 cause of death in the United States, and it's probably destined to move up the charts like a hit song, given the way we eat. It's hard to believe, but the average American scarfs down *152 pounds of sugar a year*.

It's easy to do, even if you think you're being careful. For instance, sodas contain as much as a teaspoon of sugar *per ounce*. There's sugar in catsup, salad dressing, "organic" cereals...in practically everything.

Balance your blood sugar now—*before* you get sick

We take natural supplements for cholesterol and blood pressure. Isn't it about time for a natural solution to diabetes? Jon Barron decided it was...

Seven herbs tackle diabetes seven different ways

Jon patiently pored over all the studies and competing claims for natural treatments. Ayurvedic medicine, the ancient tradition of India, alone offers 44 different herbs and formulas for diabetes. Other traditions offer dozens more.

After much study, Jon narrowed the menu down to *six* that had the best chance of creating a thorough, root-cause solution.

You thought I said *seven* herbs? I did. I'll explain about

the seventh one in a moment.

Blood sugar plummets upwards of 54 percent with one herb

The first ingredient is fenugreek. A ton of research going back to 1939 proves this herb helps control blood sugar. The herb has long been used in India, Africa and the Middle East to treat diabetes AND many other health problems as well.

In one study, researchers saw a *54% drop* in urinary glucose levels —the test doctors often use to identify diabetics.

As an added benefit, studies show <u>LDL cholesterol goes way down</u>, too.

But there's a problem—fortunately, one the researchers were able to solve.

To get the most benefit, patients had to eat a huge amount of fenugreek. The stuff tastes terrible, and as if that's not enough, it gives some people gastrointestinal side effects like gas, diarrhea or cramping.

But now a new extract concentrates the *active ingredient* in fenugreek, making much smaller doses possible and getting rid of some side effects. That's good, because...

Combine it with herb #2 and you've got a near-sure thing

During the last few years alternative doctors have given a lot of attention to gymnema sylvestre, another diabetes remedy from the Ayurvedic tradition. So naturally Jon took a close look at gymnema to see whether it lives up to the hype. It does.

It's like a dream come true for diabetics

In India they call it "the sugar destroyer." A protein in the plant not only makes you lose your craving for sugar but may actually *prevent you from digesting some of the sugar you DO eat.* It passes right through.

And here's what really got Jon Barron excited: gymnema apparently *regenerates cells in your pancreas* allowing your body to produce more insulin and helps reverse the damage diabetes does. That's the kind of root-cause solution Jon wanted to see.

In an 18-month study of gymnema, most test subjects were able to reduce their medication and some were able to get rid of drugs altogether.

Best of all, no one has reported any adverse side effects of gymnema. Not one. There are no safety issues we know of.

Just to verify Jon Barron's findings, we did some checking of our own, and we found that if you put the two herbs together you've just about got a sure thing.

Blood sugar levels plunge by more than half

You might hear of fenugreek or gymnema from other sources, but I'll bet you can't name the next five ingredients in Jon Barron's formula—much less do the hard work he did to check them out.

You'll get full details in a free Special Research Alert called ***Diabetes Defeated***. All you have to do is join Health Sciences Institute.

Even at HSI, where we hear about nearly every cure, Jon's discoveries were new to us. But, wow, do they do the job!

In one test, patients with Type II diabetes saw their fasting blood sugar levels fall an average 51.8 percent *in just 65 days*.

That's not a typo. In just a little over two months, their fasting blood sugar dropped more than half, and their levels after eating dropped an average of 84.6 percent!

Blood pressure, cholesterol and body weight drop, too

There's more. Much more. Besides the improvement in blood sugar levels, patients saw steep declines in cholesterol. Their blood pressure went down, too. In one study, participants even lost an average of 5.5 pounds.

What more could you ask?

When it comes to reducing cholesterol, researchers at the University of Toronto found that one of the herbs was more effective than some popular supplements such as oats and psyllium.

The best diabetes solution we've ever seen

Taken together in the proportions Jon figured out, the six herbs are the BEST diabetes solution we've ever seen in the eleven years since HSI was founded. A researcher told us, "It produced results that the doctors have not seen before, even with hard core drugs."

But Jon found a way to make it even better—a seventh ingredient that slashes blood sugar *and* LDL cholesterol almost 30 percent!

You see, Jon's original formula contained six herbs, but he knew there was also solid research to back the seventh ingredient—cinnamon. It just wasn't practical to include it.

That's a shame, because cinnamon *all by itself* slashes blood sugar levels AND cholesterol. In one study, participants cut their fasting glucose by 18 to 29 percent and their LDL cholesterol by 7 to 27 percent with cinnamon.

But it takes as much as a full teaspoon of cinnamon a day to do the job. That's more than Jon could pack into a supplement.

So he reluctantly left cinnamon out, till just a few months ago.

Now there's a patented cinnamon *extract*—the active ingredient—that fits in beautifully with the original formula, making a total of seven potent herbs more effective than ever before.

But you need to know more first…

As I mentioned earlier, we've arranged a discount for HSI members, and of course we'll tell the source's address, phone number and website. It's all in ***Diabetes Defeated***, a Special Research Alert we send you free as soon as you join.

Since Health Sciences Institute broke the story about Jon's formula, it's gotten so popular it practically flies off the shelves. The distributor is constantly running out, and Jon himself claims *an 82 percent success rate.*

There ARE some cautions, too, so you should read ***Diabetes Defeated*** before you take action. If you're on prescription medications—and even if you aren't—you need the guidance of a qualified health professional before you try the new remedy.

If you'd like to receive ***Diabetes Defeated***, just send in the Membership Application we enclosed. All new members also receive 7 more free reports. Better yet, join for 2 years and you get 12 free Special Research Alerts!

Chapter Five

The one-stop solution to nearly every heart problem

- Worst heart cases get better in only two weeks
- Cuts "bad" cholesterol by two-thirds
- Stops angina better than nitro – with zero side effects
- Reduces blood pressure and even promotes weight loss!

Cancel the bypass surgery?

Once in a blue moon, Health Sciences Institute uncovers a natural remedy that does so many things it's hard even for us to believe it.

But this is for real. We know that much for sure, and we can prove it with the kind of double-blind, placebo-controlled studies the medical establishment calls "the gold standard" when it comes to proof.

This "super herb" is good for more than your heart, too. We need to learn more, but it may ALSO prove to be a powerful cancer-fighter AND a potent cure for infections ranging from salmonella to pneumonia.

Remember, I'm talking about one plant. Not a formula, just *one plant*.

Bad cholesterol drops FAST

One test showed "bad" LDL cholesterol plunged an average of 25.6 percent after a mere 30 days on the supplement. The control group's cholesterol didn't change a bit.

But that's nothing! *In another test, bad cholesterol levels went down two-thirds in 60 days!*

What's more, the herb has NO adverse side effects. It's totally safe. That means you could get out of the statin drug trap once and for all.

If you're on statin drugs or your doctor is bugging you about your cholesterol, you've GOT to check this out. We'll send you all the details in a Special Report called *The Secret Cures for Heart Disease*—yours free when you become a member of Health Sciences Institute.

Equals prescription drugs for angina, slashes angina episodes by half

The herbal remedy is a godsend for more than six million Americans who suffer from angina. These folks experience frightening chest pains that can make them think they're having a heart attack.

The most common prescription drug for angina is nitroglycerin. But nitro has a major drawback: Each time you use it nitro is less effective. I'd say that's a problem.

And if that's not bad enough, nitro can also cause lightheadedness, dizziness, a rapid pulse, and blurred vision.

A distinguished foreign medical school investigated

and found that the herbal remedy <u>outperformed nitro in a head-to-head test</u>. Even more exciting, the herbal remedy had NO side effects. NONE at all.

And unlike nitroglycerin, the herbal remedy doesn't lose its power over time. It works as well the last time you use it as the first.

In another study, <u>the number of angina episodes went down by half</u>. Better yet, the test participants <u>lowered their blood pressure</u> and even <u>lost a bit of weight</u>.

What more can you ask? Well, actually, a lot more...

Most severe heart cases improve in two weeks

Patients suffering from congestive heart failure are classified into four groups, ranging from mild to severe. Those in the worst group, class IV, are darn near hopeless.

In a study of the herb, <u>class IV patients improved so quickly they were reclassified as class III in only two weeks</u>.

And what is this natural wonder? Something new from a supplement maker eager to make a buck? Not at all! It's another gift from India's 2,700-year-old tradition of Ayurvedic medicine.

Yup! People have been using this stuff for almost 3,000 years—*safely and effectively*.

How on earth can medical science ignore this?

Good question. The answer is, the system is geared to making money, and there's no money in a natural remedy, even one that's proven effective for almost 3,000 years.

If a plant remedy can't be patented, it may as well be grass clippings from your lawn. If there's no patent, the drug company can't own all the rights and reap billions.

Next time you're in a library, just look at a medical journal, the kind doctors read to keep up with new developments. Almost all the ads are from big drug companies.

And maybe it's not obvious, but most of the "editorial" content reports the results of studies on—you guessed it— pharmaceutical drugs. And the studies are funded by— you guessed it—the drug companies.

In other words, basically ALL medical literature is funded and created by drug companies. What they call "continuing education" in the medical profession is a suc- cession of drug company ads—some actually labeled "ads" and some labeled "scientific research."

Cholesterol drops 78 points in a month!

"I just had to e-mail you and let you know how much you have saved me from having to be on Zocor!!! Besides being a prescription drug and costing over $150 per month, it was not lowering my cholesterol. Then one day in your Alert, I read about [your herbal solution]...In one month's time my cholesterol lowered from 277 to 199!"

F.B., Member

It's a closed circle, and you won't get out of it unless you take yourself out of it

Every month Health Sciences Institute brings you breaking news on alternative treatments and nutrients your doctor will never see in the publications he or she reads. Often, we're the first to discover and publicize new alternative health solutions. In fact, we're usually the first.

As soon as you join, we'll send you all the information you need about the Ayurvedic heart remedy from India, plus other heart and stroke solutions, in your free Special Research Alert, *The Secret Cures for Heart Disease*.

Just mail us the Membership Application enclosed with this book.

My "desert island" answer to heart failure

There are so many different natural solutions for everything from cancer to heart disease to pain to allergies...

Friends often ask me which is the best one—the one I'd have to have if I were stuck on a desert island.

If I thought I was at risk for heart attack or stroke, it's no contest.

My choice would be a super-potent enzyme found in a cheese-like Japanese food called natto, made from fermented soybeans. The supplement is called "nattokinase," which just means "natto enzyme."

The reason is that heart attacks and most strokes occur when a blood clot closes off a blood vessel. If the blood vessel goes to your brain, you suffer a stroke. If it goes to your heart, you have a heart attack. If you can dissolve the clot quickly, the problem is over.

Have you heard you should take an aspirin if you think you're having a heart attack? They tell you that because aspirin is a *blood thinner*. It will help break up the clot.

Mother nature does it better

Aspirin is better than nothing, but *nattokinase* —the enzyme I'm talking about—is probably the most potent clot-buster on earth, natural or synthetic according to in vivo studies. If you're lucky enough to get to an ER, they MIGHT give you a clot-busting drug (cost: $20,000 per dose). But they probably won't. Many hospitals don't even have it in stock.

Besides, nattokinase is more powerful. As often happens, a natural substance outperforms any product the big drug companies have come up with. What's more, natto has been tested and proven effective upwards of an hour. Compare that to the $20K stuff, which peters out in less than 20 minutes. But most important, you can take nattokinase at home at the first sign of a problem.

It could become the biggest heart breakthrough in history

The natto story is unfolding even as I write this. It may turn out to be the best all around heart, cholesterol, blood-pressure and plaque-fighting remedy ever found.

Early human and animal tests already show it slashes blood pressure within days and it might even dissolve the deadly plaque that lines arteries.

But even though nattokinase is a natural remedy—it's a powerful one. So you shouldn't mix it with prescription heart, stroke or blood pressure drugs. Consult a qualified health professional about whether nattokinase is right for you. And keep an eye on future issues of our Health Sciences Institute newsletter for breaking news about this natural miracle.

WE SCOOPED 'EM ALL...

Health Sciences Institute was the first to break the exciting news about nattokinase, in our March, 2000 issue. Back then, you couldn't even get the stuff in the U.S.

So you've got a clear choice when it comes to alternatives: You can wait a year or two until someone else copies our latest discovery. Or you can wait 5 or 6 years till the mainstream press picks it up. Or you can wait up to 17 years for a drug company to patent an imitation and charge a fortune for it.

Or you can join the 90,000 doctors, scientists, health practitioners and informed citizens who belong to Health Sciences Institute—and be the first to get the latest breakthrough.

43

Tuna extract beats blood pressure drugs?

Your free report on forbidden heart cures also features a new blood pressure breakthrough—the Asian bonito fish, a relative of the tuna family. But I don't mean you should eat the fish. In fact, that won't do you any good.

For 1,500 years, the Japanese have used the fish to make a highly-prized traditional seasoning—and the new blood pressure remedy is actually made from the <u>residue they used to throw away after making the sauce</u>! One man's trash turned out to be another man's treasure.

A Japanese doctor learned he could separate, purify and ferment these valuable fish proteins into an extract that relaxes blood vessels. Clinical tests prove it's better than expensive ACE-inhibiting drugs. What's more, the fish extract is cheaper AND safer.

This may be the most powerful answer to blood pressure yet! Learn more in your FREE report, *The Secret Cures for Heart Disease*.

The Secret Cures for

HEART DISEASE

**One of 8
Special Research Alerts
for New Members**

Chapter Six

Fix 12 years of memory loss...and stop Alzheimer's dead in its tracks?!

Patients with the most damage see the greatest improvement

And it's not just people with advanced cases who can benefit. These breakthroughs could help ANYONE who needs a memory boost—and who doesn't? I don't mind saying my own memory isn't what it used to be!

That's exactly how Alzheimer's begins. It's a long slide down to a very dark place, a place where you can't even recognize your own family or remember your own name.

DON'T SIT BY QUIETLY...
We now have the tools to stop it

Learn about how Thomas Crooks co-wrote the landmark study on a memory supplement that was published in the medical journal *Neurology*. He says that researchers noted that in one way in particular it was as if the supplement...

"may reverse approximately 12 years of decline"

He's talking about a *food*—for crying out loud. It's an essential fatty acid called Phosphatidyl serine, or PS.

In a study of folks over 50 with memory loss, Crooks and his colleagues saw dramatic memory improvement take place in only 12 weeks. *Amazingly, those with the most memory loss enjoyed the greatest benefit.*

PS is just one of a bagful of mind-saving miracles I'll tell you about in the next two minutes. But how come you never hear about these breakthroughs in the United States? Let me answer you by saying...

"Dear FDA: We can't wait 17 years when the answers are here now"

We're in the midst of a national crisis. Our nursing homes are already packed with tragic Alzheimer's victims.

Meanwhile, the evidence that we can SOLVE ALZHEIMER'S is so impressive, folks are snapping up these natural remedies like a hot Internet stock—<u>everywhere in the world except here</u>.

One of the natural cures is used in 15 European countries and is backed by dozens of clinical studies on thousands of patients.

But when it comes to natural remedies, U.S. drug companies won't spend a single penny of their billions—which they get from us, after all.

Maybe they think they can cook up a synthetic version of these treatments, but why should we wait 17 years? That's the typical amount of time it takes for important research to trickle down to doctors and hospitals, according to a study by the National Academy of Sciences.

Mountains of red tape and bureaucratic nonsense keep

us from getting the treatments we need, not just PS, but others, too. Here's how to free yourself from their tyranny...

Most people get better in only four weeks— at a cost of pennies per day

For centuries, an extract of *Chinese club moss* has been used in traditional Chinese medicine to treat fever and inflammation. Chinese scientists had a hunch it might help people with memory loss, too. And boy, were they right!

One study of 202 patients suffering from age-related memory loss showed *after only four weeks, 70 percent of those tested showed improvement in cognitive function and quality of life. <u>Seven out of ten</u>*.

The plant extract not only stopped memory loss, it reversed it!

Now a professor of pharmacology at Georgetown University admits the Chinese herb "may actually slow the progression of Alzheimer's disease." The Georgetown researchers declare the extract may be...

Superior to the leading drugs approved for treating Alzheimer's

What's more, we have a pretty good idea of why the plant extract works. In Alzheimer's, a body chemical called AchE runs amok and destroys a vital neurotransmitter called acetylcholine, or AC.

How important is AC? VERY. If you're able to read this, you can thank your healthy levels of AC.

As we age, our AC levels go down naturally. But in Alzheimer's, something goes horribly wrong, and the brain tissue that produces AC is the first tissue to be destroyed.

Scientists know that in advanced Alzheimer's patients, AC levels plunge by 90 percent.

> *If you can hang on to your AC, you can hang on to your memory.* **This is NOT quack medicine. It's good science, accepted by mainstream and alternative doctors alike.**

The Georgetown team AND researchers at an Israeli institute found the club moss extract specifically inhibits AchE, the bad chemical in your brain that destroys your AC.

Result: you can remember where you left your keys

You'll learn everything you need to know when you join Health Sciences Institute. It's all in a free Special Research Alert we send to every new member, *Stop Memory Loss Dead in its Tracks*.

The Research Alert reveals no less than three exciting solutions to memory loss. We show you how to order the club moss extract. What's more, the club moss formula combines the herb with six other brain boosters.

One of these powerful supplements is alpha-lipoic acid or ALA, proven by a German study to stop Alzheimer's cold. The patients who take ALA stop sliding downhill. Period.

The formula also features PS, the essential fatty acid I

mentioned at the beginning of this chapter. More than two dozen clinical trials confirm the power of PS to improve learning and memory. But even PS may pale compared to...

The most powerful, most widely accepted memory supplement

Health Sciences Institute recently broke the story of what may be the most exciting Alzheimer's treatment yet. If you like to garden, you may know it as one of the first flowers to bloom every spring. Now, these nodding little white bells may deliver us from a dreaded disease, once and for all.

I'm talking about *snowdrops*. They got their name because sometimes they come up right through the snow.

What a lovely symbol for the new life they can bring our minds!

Call it springtime for your brain

The snowdrop extract <u>totally halted the loss of mental ability</u> in five studies involving 3,000 Belgian patients. *The people on the extract held their own or got better*, while those on a placebo continued to slide downhill, as you'd expect with Alzheimer's.

Other studies, including one at the University of Rochester, demonstrated the same miraculous healing.

You don't have to wait for the cure

Dozens of recent clinical trials show the snowdrop extract beats all the prescription Alzheimer's drugs. Even the boneheads at the FDA have been forced to pay heed.

But I wouldn't wait around while they think about it for 17 years. The snowdrop extract is accepted in 15 European countries, and you can benefit today.

Our researchers describe this remedy, and the other memory-savers I've mentioned, in detail—with everything you need to know—in your free copy of ***Stop Memory Loss Dead in its Tracks***. Send for yours today. We enclosed a Membership Application for you.

Chapter Seven

Beyond pain killers:
A real answer to arthritis

**Reduces joint swelling by 97 percent...and outper-
forms next-best natural remedy by 200-to-one!**

Dear arthritis sufferer, your life sentence to pain killers
has just been commuted. Read this chapter and you're free
to go—without pills.

And not a moment too soon! NO prescription or
over-the-counter pain reliever is totally safe. NOT ONE.
All have toxic side effects, up to and including death. And
death is a pretty serious side effect.

Did you know that "harmless" anti-inflammatory drugs
like aspirin and ibuprofen send more than 100,000 people a
year to the hospital with gastrointestinal bleeding? More
than 16,000 of these poor folks die. These over-the-counter
painkillers are a leading cause of ulcers.

The number one cause of liver failure
is a pain reliever

How about acetaminophen, the active ingredient in
Tylenol? The good news: It doesn't hurt your stomach. The
bad news: It's one of the leading causes of liver failure.

I hope you read the labels VERY carefully and take

ONLY as directed. They aren't kidding.

Of course, reading the warnings doesn't always help. Remember Vioxx, the pain-killing wonder drug touted in millions of dollars' worth of feel-good TV commercials? It got yanked off the market. Turns out Vioxx nearly DOUBLED your risk of stroke and heart attack. And the manufacturer, uh, knew but sort of neglected to tell us.

Pain relief is great, but now you can get more

We've found potent *natural* pain relievers that are totally safe, and cheap, too! You'll learn some of the best in a free Special Research Alert entitled *Pain Free for Life*.

But the Holy Grail of alternative medicine was something more, much more, than just masking pain. Researchers the world over looked high and low for a safe, natural remedy that would target the root cause of arthritis and get rid of it once and for all.

You see, our whole purpose is to solve your problem, not to keep you coming back every week for the rest of your life to buy more pills. So let me tell you about another Health Sciences Institute first...

Find out who's healthy and ask why

In alternative health, a good rule of thumb is to look at people who are healthy and figure out why. Then do whatever it is they're doing.

That's especially true when a WHOLE NATIVE POPULATION is healthy and doesn't have some disease that's an epidemic in developed countries like ours.

That's how alternative health researchers found out about omega-3 fatty acids. Now we know that these natural oils found in salmon and other cold water fish are vital to a healthy heart and arteries.

It's all because someone was smart enough to ask, "What makes people healthy?" instead of just asking, "What cures people who are sick?"

When researchers began to look at it that way, they noticed that the native Inuit people or "Eskimos" were almost totally free of cardiovascular disease. They suffered almost no strokes, heart attacks, hardening of the arteries, or high cholesterol.

Lo and behold, it turns out the Eskimos' high-fish diet was extremely rich in omega-3's, and now millions of us benefit from omega-3 supplements.

New Zealand's natives don't get arthritis

When researchers tried the same approach to arthritis, the native population that stood out was the Maori of New Zealand, especially those who dwell on the coast of that island paradise.

Researchers noticed the Maori hardly ever get arthritis. Even into their 70s, 80s and 90s, their joints remain supple and pain-free. According to one amazed writer, an elderly Maori can scamper and climb like a teenager at an age when most Americans need a cane, a walker or a wheelchair.

The secret is a gourmet delicacy

It was a challenge to figure out what specific food held the key to such vitality, but the Maori's own stories contained a clue. According to a centuries-old tradition, eating a shellfish called *the green-lipped mussel* leads to a long and healthy life.

It wasn't easy to confirm the legend. In fact, it took decades of research by dedicated scientists. By 1980, they knew enough to conduct a double-blind, placebo-controlled trial on arthritis patients in the UK. These folks had failed to respond to conventional treatment and were scheduled for joint surgery.

Back then, the scientists didn't know WHAT was in the mussel that might cure joint disease. So they made a powdered supplement out of the whole thing.

The patients assigned to the placebo group experienced no improvement and had to go ahead with their surgery. But it was a different story indeed for the group that took powdered mussel. <u>76% of the patients with rheumatoid arthritis got better and so did 70% percent of those with osteoarthritis</u>.

Your choice: 70 percent healthier or 30 percent sicker

It's a fact. Even in this early test, people with *both* types of arthritis got better!

Remember, none of these patients knew whether they

were receiving the mussel extract or a sugar pill. All they knew for sure was how much pain they felt. That's why studies like this are called "double-blind."

18-year multinational effort seeks the cure

This all sounds easy when described in a few paragraphs, but in fact the research continued for 18 years, led by top scientists from universities and labs in Australia, Japan and France. But not in America. If you've read this far, you know why.

Hot on the trail of the sea critter's unknown "active ingredient," their excitement mounted as each phase yielded a more powerful compound. <u>Even early versions were found to be more effective than aspirin and ibuprofen in reducing inflammation</u>.

The Maori secret stands revealed

Now we DO know the "secret ingredient," thanks to their determined efforts. And here's something really fascinating: the secret is a unique configuration of fatty acids called ETA's. They're actually related to omega-3's like those found in salmon.

But "unique" means unique: The grouping of fatty acids found in New Zealand's green-lipped mussel is found nowhere else on earth, as far as science can tell.

Once they identified the fatty acid, researchers worked fast to prove the amazing arthritis-fighting properties of this rare seafood product. In animal experiments, joint swelling from arthritis was <u>reduced by 93 percent</u>.

And in humans the results were even more astounding. In one double-blind study, the patented green-lipped mussel extract was <u>nearly 100 percent effective in humans</u> (97 percent, to be precise).

What's more, the natural remedy has NO known adverse side effects.

Hundreds of times more powerful than other natural remedies

Alternative healers have known for years that natural lipids or fatty acids help reduce inflammation and reduce arthritis pain. If you suffer from arthritis, you may already take flaxseed oil, evening primrose oil, Norwegian salmon oil, or Max EPA (a high-potency fish oil product).

Tests show the green-lipped mussel extract outperforms them all—and by such a crushing margin there's no contest. The mussel extract reduced arthritis-related swelling by 79 percent.

Another historic "first" for natural medicine

The scientists received a patent for their discovery. That's rare for a natural cure. But in this case it was more than justified by the huge effort it took to identify and isolate this medical miracle. It could be one of the most important therapies ever to emerge from alternative medicine.

You'll want all the details for yourself and everyone you know who suffers from the pain and swelling of arthritis. It's all in a Special Research Alert called ***Pain Free for Life***—rushed to you with our compliments when you become a member of Health Sciences Institute.

And remember, you get a total of 8 free Research Alerts (12 with a two-year membership) —plus our monthly newsletter and many other privileges.

You can join today by mailing your Membership Application. We enclosed a loose one with this book. But if you misplaced it, you'll find an extra copy at the end of this book.

Chapter Eight

A rare prostate herb so powerful... The growers want to keep it all for themselves!

But we've found a source. Keep reading...

Our source claims that 16 men with advanced prostate cancer were totally cured. And hundreds of patients prove almost 100% success in treating enlarged prostate.

P.S. It's good for women, too!

If you're tired of supplement makers who try to sell you some new herbal cure for sky-high prices—here's a refreshing change:

The Asian country that grows this prostate herb wants to keep every ounce of it for the home market! That's how good it is. At one time, it was even reserved for the royal family and called "Medicine for the King's Palace."

The country I'm thinking of is Vietnam, and that's a name you don't hear often in the world of alternative medicine. You should—and you will—because a couple of years ago Health Sciences Institute began to research and publish the best of Vietnam's rich legacy of traditional medicine.

Our first discovery was another HSI first in North

America. It's a remarkable plant proven to clear up the symptoms of enlarged prostate in *92.6 percent of the men* who try it. I'm not talking about anecdotal cases involving one or two men. No way!

144 out of 149 men cured of BPH?! Can you believe it? How are they hiding this from us?

If you're a male of a certain age, you probably know about enlarged prostate, also called benign prostatic hyperplasia or BPH.

If you suffer from BPH you feel like "you've gotta go" over and over again—especially at night, when you're trying to get some sleep. Sometimes urination is painful, and often the stream is weak and interrupted because the swollen prostate shuts off the tube—called the urethra— that the urine flows through.

If those symptoms sound familiar, a free Special Research Alert called *The Powerful Prostate Antidote* could be the answer to your prayers. Health Sciences Institute will rush you a copy as soon as you become a member. We enclosed a loose application for you and you'll find extras at the end of the book.

Join us today! Because there's more...

BPH is bad enough, but you can live with it, and millions of men do. Not so when it comes to the most dreaded prostate problem—cancer. Prostate tumors are so common you're just about sure to get them if you live long enough.

The Vietnamese "Medicine for the King's Palace" has

been highly successful in TOTALLY CURING PROSTATE CANCER. It's the absolute truth. In one study, 16 men with *advanced* prostate cancer were completely cured. Biopsies confirmed it. And American cancer victims will tell you the same thing...

An American with a special interest in prostate cancer got wind of the Vietnamese remedy and tried it himself.

You see, Ken Malik, the guy I'm talking about, was not only a prostate cancer victim but he actually co-founded and ran the Prostate Awareness Foundation, a non-profit group based in San Francisco.

Ken had enjoyed some success over an eight-year period with a popular remedy called PC Spes. You may have heard about PC Spes because it got a lot of press. But it was pulled off the market when it was found to contain non-natural and possibly harmful ingredients.

The PC Spes fiasco turned out to be good luck for Ken!

Suddenly left without a treatment he thought he needed for his prostate cancer, Ken scrambled for a replacement. He found the Vietnamese herbal. <u>And after just ten months on the remedy, a biopsy indicated his prostate was completely free of cancer cells!</u>

Ken was so excited he organized his own test with ten fellow members of the Prostate Awareness Foundation. After only three months all of them experienced improvement.

In one case, a 58-year-old man's PSA count was an

astronomical 93. (A reading of less than four is considered normal.) That's enough to scare the daylights out of most guys, and in this case the fear was well-founded. Tests revealed the man's cancer had spread to his bones, intestines and lymph nodes.

A conventional medical doctor would have told the man to make out his will.

Instead, the "terminal case" went on an aggressive herbal program that included the Vietnamese prostate herb. *In only four months his PSA was down to 0.9.* That's not a misprint—his PSA score was *less than one*. What's more, many of his disease symptoms disappeared. To put it plainly, he felt better.

It's hard to get, but HSI found a way

The herb is so popular as a prostate AND ovarian treatment in Vietnam, the government forbids exporting it. They want to keep this precious substance for their own citizens.

Not to worry. Health Sciences Institute located an exclusive source. Because the supply is so limited, we must share the information only with our members. But you'll receive everything you need to know in the free report. We have no connection to any supplement company and we don't profit from your decision.

To find out more, send in the Membership Application enclosed with this book (there are extras on the last few pages, too).

Chapter Nine

100% success in treating cataracts without drugs or surgery

For a nickel a day you may never worry again about losing your vision...

If you develop cataracts, the choice is either surgery or blindness, right? Not anymore.

While American doctors perform one-and-a-half million cataract surgeries a year (and then have to repeat half of those because the cataracts come back)...

European doctors have developed *safe, natural eye drops* that work to clear up your vision in a matter of months without surgery.

What's more, this easy answer has been around for years. The eye drops have even been featured on European TV. In a sort of "reality TV" experiment, four people, including one of the show's hosts, actually tried the product. The idea was to see if it lived up to the claims.

Did it ever!

The show created a sensation in Britain and led many people to try the new eye drops.

"Five years ago I was told I must not drive..."

...wrote one British resident. "Two years ago I was

warned that the cataracts were just about fully formed and I needed check-ups every six months...I have now been using carnosine eye drops for six months. I recently went to the optician and was told I only had a bit of a cataract. Also, I do not need to see an optician for two years. I could not believe it..."

Why haven't you heard about this astonishing breakthrough? Maybe because it's a threat to a multi billion dollar branch of the American medical business: cataract surgery.

A few drops a day, cataracts go away?

"In October, 2002, I was diagnosed with a small cataract in my left eye," writes M.S. in England. "Shortly afterwards a work colleague told me about the eye drops, as seen on channel 4 'Richard & Judy.' I started using them. In April, 2004, I had an in-depth eye test: NO SIGN OF THE CATARACT."

These Brits cleared up their vision problem with just a few drops in each eye, several times a day. But I've got even better news for you...

You can use the drops to help *prevent* cataracts, too!

And the sooner you get started, the better! The lens of your eye is more permeable in the early stages, before the cataracts become advanced. For prevention, the maker recommends just one or two drops in each eye once a day.

Cost? About a nickel a day. Maybe a dime.

The secret is a natural body chemical called N-acetyl

L-carnosine—or NAC, for short—combined with selected antioxidants in a special formula.

A brilliant European biochemist developed the breakthrough after his own father got cataracts. Before his dad developed a problem, this professor had been studying another form of carnosine without even thinking about eye health.

But when he saw what was happening to his father, he remembered some research he'd seen indicating that NAC could help treat cataracts.

Turned out it wasn't that simple, and the scientist had to spend years researching and developing a NAC-based formula that could knock out cataracts with a simple course of eye drops.

The solution arrived too late for the scientist's father— he had to have surgery anyway. But it could be just in time for YOU if you're starting to have vision problems.

How this miracle works

If you know anything about health, it won't surprise you to learn that free radicals are the main culprits that make our eyes age—in fact, free radicals are a key reason that ALL our tissues age. You may also know that antioxidants such as vitamin A and vitamin E fight free radicals and help prevent disease and aging.

Free radical damage to our eyes can come from pollution, diabetes, smoking, poor diet, ultraviolet rays from sunlight, and many other sources. Our bodies are under assault every second of every day from free radical attackers.

Our eyes are especially vulnerable to free radical damage that causes clumping or cross-linking of proteins. Cross-linking causes the lenses of your eyes to become clouded.

Think of it like cooking an egg white. It's clear and fluid as it hits the pan, but the heat causes the proteins to cross-link. The egg changes from clear and fluid to white and rubbery. That's roughly what free radicals and aging do to your eyes.

Getting the antioxidants into your eye tissue is a problem

Alternative health experts know that antioxidants can fight free radical damage in the eye. Your mailbox may be full of offers for "new" or "special" or "breakthrough" antioxidants such as bilberry that are said to help your eyes. And some of them can do just that.

Studies prove a vitamin E solution in your eyes helps repair tissues and even prevents cataracts from forming in the first place.

The problem is, our eyes and lenses are very imperme-able. They keep out topical liquids like a raincoat. But NAC—the breakthrough ingredient in the new eye drops dissolves in fats AND water.

That means NAC penetrates the eye's lens and delivers a powerful antioxidant that reverses the cross-linking process that makes the lens cloudy.

Once in your eyes, NAC breaks down into L-carnosine —

a powerful antioxidant in itself. But it does even more: it turns out NAC is a powerful *delivery vehicle* for other antioxidants such as A and E. These natural substances are like a healing balm to your eyes—IF you can get them to penetrate the lens.

And that's exactly what the NAC formula does.

Every single patient got better

A 1999 Chinese study achieved 100 percent success on early-stage, old-age-related cataracts.

That's right: 100 percent. Every single patient got better. But here's something even more amazing...

The study showed 80 percent success against ADVANCED cataracts, too!

Meanwhile, a double-blind, placebo-controlled study in Russia confirmed the same thing the Chinese doctors witnessed. <u>In the Russian study, vision improved in 90 percent of the patients who received a NAC formula, and none of the patients got worse</u>.

Among the folks on a placebo, it was a different story! 89 percent of them experienced *worse vision* by the end of the study.

So what do you want? A 90 percent chance of getting better or an 89 percent chance of getting worse?

If this was a prescription drug, they'd yell at you for NOT taking it!

If this was a prescription drug, a sales rep would call

on your doctor every week and try to get him to prescribe it for you. Instead, it's a cheap, natural remedy. No corporation is going to spend billions to educate your doctor about it. No way! If anything, they'll spend billions lying about it and keeping it away from you.

Meanwhile, doctors hardly ever get sued for botched cataract surgery. They don't have to worry about controversy. The insurance companies pay for surgery without a quibble. The patients usually go along because the surgery

---

Powerful new answer to macular degeneration

Macular degeneration is an even greater threat to your vision than cataracts, and much harder to treat. In fact, age related macular degeneration (ARMD) is the leading cause of blindness.

At Health Sciences Institute, we've been on the lookout for an ARMD answer for a long time. *This is the first promising discovery we've found.*

If you know anything about eye health, you're probably aware of lutein. It's one of a powerful family of antioxidants that can cross the blood-brain barrier and benefit your eyes. But this new nutrient goes...

Beyond lutein

Now we've located a member of the same antioxidant family that may be the most potent ARMD treatment ever. It's a substance, actually a pigment, found in certain

is "minor."

For the medical industry, it's like a dream! Problem is, it's not a patient's dream. You don't need someone taking a knife to your eyes if it's totally unnecessary.

Find out for yourself, with all the details on the eye drops, in a free Special Research Alert called *Vital Health Secrets*. There's a Membership Application at the end of the book.

---

varieties of algae. In fact, pink-tinted sea creatures such as salmon and shrimp actually get their color from eating these algae.

But it's just about impossible for you to eat enough of the right seafood to get the dose you need.

Instead, researchers in Korea and at Japan's National Institute of Health and Nutrition focused on extracting the nutrient from the algae itself. <u>The result is an antioxidant twice as effective as beta-carotene</u>

<u>and nearly 80 times more effective than vitamin E</u>.

And as I mentioned, it crosses the blood-brain barrier and bathes your eyes in nutrients. Only a very special, limited number of antioxidants can do this.

When it comes to macular degeneration, this is it. We'll provide you with full details in a free Special Research Alert, *Vital Health Secrets*. Just send in the Membership Application at the end of this book.

Chapter Ten

Control your bladder the natural way

Dear Corporate America,
You can keep your overpriced diapers...

If you've seen those TV ads for Depends and similar products, you might wonder what our "golden years" have in store for us. Will we have to have worry about our bladders every minute?

No way!

At Health Sciences Institute, we're convinced that nature has an answer for everything our bodies need. That includes a healthy bladder. Now, thanks to one of our distinguished HSI panelists, Dr. Allen N. Spreen, we can bring our members...

Another Health Sciences Institute First

When Dr. Spreen tells us he's got important news, we listen. He's an M.D. and one of the heavy hitters on our Advisory Panel. That's saying something, because every member of our panel is a star in the world of alternative medicine.

Dr. Spreen has not only helped thousands of patients in his private practice, but he's also helped *millions* through TV's Discovery Channel, America Online's natural health website, and his trailblazing books on nutrition.

One of his books, *Nutritionally Incorrect*, has been

called the Bible of sound nutrition.

A few months ago, Dr. Spreen told us he and his team had found a natural solution to bladder health. You can bet we stopped the presses and rushed the news to our members! What's the big deal? If you've ever had your bladder control your day, you darn well know…

Every day can be an emergency

And if you think it's not an "emergency," you've never been hit with that terrible "oops" experience—without warning—at a party, or on the golf course, or in church. No matter where it happens, one thing's for sure—it's ALWAYS a bad time!

Of course the usual corporate types are rushing to cash in with band-aid solutions that keep you coming back to the store every week to plunk down your money. We knew there had to be a better way.

Most solutions are "all wet"

Dr. Spreen and his team of researchers combed the world's scientific and medical literature to find EVERY herb, mineral, vitamin or other nutrient that's said to improve bladder health.

Then they really got down to work.

They *evaluated* each of these alternative foods and remedies. But they found most of them don't have what it takes.

That's okay. You don't need dozens of remedies, you just

need one or two that work. And out of that long list of possibilities, Dr. Spreen's team finally found the herbal answers.

An ancient solution for your bladder

Under the common name *three-leaf caper*, the first herb has been renowned for centuries in the Ayurvedic tradition of India. Yes, this 2,700-year-old body of medical knowledge has produced yet another breakthrough.

The ground-up bark of this Himalayan tree is so highly regarded for its healing properties that it's often grown near places of worship. That's why the tree's botanical name is *Crateva religiosa*.

I can tell you this for sure: A lot of our readers thank God for the relief!

The second herb, horsetail, is found closer to home. It's known to soothe the lining of the urinary tract. More than that, the researchers found it reduces muscle spasms and supports the sphincters that give us voluntary control.

This formula lets *you* decide when to go!

Both herbs are available in a single, proprietary preparation available from only one source. We'll tell you all about it in a free Special Research Alert called *Control Your Bladder the Natural Way*.

If you join HSI as a new member, we'll rush you a copy right away.

I could go on all day about the remarkable power of

these herbs...the way they can give you back control of your life and let you socialize or enjoy sports and other activities...how you can sleep all night without getting up to go...and how you'll make fewer trips to the bathroom during the day.

There isn't enough space here, so get the free report. Just send in a Membership Application form the end of the book, or the loose one we enclosed in the envelope. We included a postage-paid envelope, too!

For a full summary of membership privileges, including up to TWELVE free Special Research Alerts, see Chapter 17, page 105.

Chapter Eleven

The "missing link" in your energy level

...is a rare nutrient now available in supplement form for the first time

The only "drawback" might be *too much* energy... but you can always cut back on this food!

P.S. It's good for your heart, too.

If you want a rocket to take off, it makes sense to fill it with rocket fuel, don't you think? You don't pull up to a gas station and fill it with unleaded regular.

Your body's rocket fuel is a substance called ATP, an enzyme inside each and every cell that makes it go. If you want to boost your energy at the cellular level, you've got to get your ATP levels up.

The <u>real</u> reason you feel tired all the time

The problem is, it's not easy to boost your ATP. Our bodies make ATP in a complex, multi-step process that just plain fails to work in many of us. ATP levels can fall as we get older or if we suffer from heart disease, fibromyalgia or a whole range of other conditions.

<u>One of the body's critical building blocks for ATP is a certain rare type of sugar</u>.

This sugar is <u>not</u> the stuff on your table, much less the corn-syrup junk that corporate food giants put in sodas and other processed foods (with our government's blessing.) What's more, this type of sugar does no harm to diabetics. In fact...

The sugar you need is not found in any food!
Your body has to make its own.

The sugar your body needs is called *ribose*. Your body can make ribose naturally, but it takes several enzymes, and those enzymes are lacking in your heart and muscle cells.

Worse yet, <u>no</u> foods contain ribose in any substantial amounts. But when our hearts or muscles are exhausted, they *need* ribose to make ATP. I'd call that a problem. No wonder so many of us·are tired all the time!

Another Health Sciences Institute "first"

Now there's an answer—from Hyla Cass, an M.D. who serves on our distinguished Health Sciences Institute Advisory Panel.

At HSI we're so used to high-powered doctors and scientists that we get a little blasé about them—but not about Dr. Cass!

She's an Assistant Clinical Professor at the world-renowned UCLA School of Medicine. She's also written a shelf-full of books such as *8 Weeks to Vibrant Health: A Woman's Take-Charge Program to Correct Imbalances, Reclaim Energy and Restore Well-Being.*

Get your energy answer from an energy expert

Dr. Cass is a renowned national authority on energy and chronic fatigue. She's always on the lookout for ways to tackle this hard-to-treat problem, so she was really excited when she came across the new discovery.

The breakthrough is actually in the manufacturing process. This is a case of high tech working hand in hand with natural medicine. You see, even though ribose is seldom found in food, supplement makers *can* synthesize it in a lab—but only at very great expense.

Until now, that is. The new discovery makes it possible to manufacture ribose inexpensively. Anyone who needs a lift can afford it.

The new supplement is *chemically identical* to the ribose your own body makes. And early results show the supplement can work *virtual miracles*—even in the hardest cases of fatigue.

I guess she follows her own energy advice because she's a one-woman ball of fire! Somehow she finds time for charitable work with Vitamin Relief USA, a nonprofit group that provides daily supplements to children in need.

Wipe out pain and fatigue in two weeks

The hardest cases of chronic pain are caused by fibromyalgia—a form of chronic fatigue and pain that has scientists totally stumped. No one knows what causes it, but it can reduce vibrant young people to near-invalids who can't climb a flight of stairs.

Dr. Cass relates the story of Kris, a veterinary surgeon and researcher at a major university. At age 37, this accomplished woman had to give up her work after fibromyalgia hit her. The disease had ruined her life.

But then a wonderful thing happened...

Kris started supplementing with ribose and felt better within ONE WEEK. And within six weeks she was close to feeling like her old self again. But the *real proof* is what happened when she stopped taking ribose. She quickly became debilitated again, lost all the function she had regained and the pain returned too. That's until Kris returned to...

Nature's astonishing "Miracle Sugar"

Dr. Cass also reports amazing results in people with heart problems. Extra ribose can offset the energy drain that often goes along with congestive heart failure, artery disease and related heart conditions.

What's more, it's not just a matter of relieving fatigue. The new supplement may actually help *reverse* heart disease, because low ATP and ribose can starve the heart of oxygen.

Can healthy folks benefit from ribose supplements? Absolutely! Dr. Cass says athletes can take up to 5 grams to supercharge their workouts. That's about one teaspoon. Even couch potatoes can benefit from low doses of ribose.

And how about safety?

You'll be happy to know you can mix ribose safely with any medication. Thousands of patients have taken it. There are <u>no side effects</u> even at 60 grams (a whopping 60,000 milligrams) a day. And that's *twelve times* the recommended supplement of five grams per day.

Think about it. Your body makes ribose naturally and it works with your body's own chemistry. What harm can the supplement possibly do? The jackbooted thugs at the FDA will have a hard time coming up with scare stories about this one.

Okay, there may be ONE side effect...

Dr. Cass says, "The only warning I give patients is that it may cause over-stimulation if taken too close to bedtime. In that case, I recommend that they take it earlier in the day."

If you want more energy, I bet that's a chance you're willing to take!

To find out more, just become a member of Health Sciences Institute. We'll rush you a FREE copy of our Special Research Alert, *Natural Energy Boosters.*

As you know, we have no connection with any supplement company. We don't profit if you decide to try this remarkable nutrient. Our only mission is to help you get better.

Mail us the loose Membership Application we enclosed, or one of the extras bound into the end of this book. You'll get the energy report and seven others. Or join for two years and get all TWELVE FREE RESEARCH ALERTS—a full library of rare, forbidden and banned alternative cures.

Can you afford to be without this information?

Almost every cure I've mentioned in this book is an HSI first—our members knew about them before anyone else. The medical establishment has successfully kept this information out of our country, so even alternative doctors often don't know. Or they know, and they're afraid to tell you for fear of losing their licenses!

Make sure *you're* in the loop! Get the full collection of free Special Research Alerts—plus your monthly issues of our newsletter AND our daily e-mails.

Chapter Twelve

Worst leukemia victim in 20 years gets well

...with a natural cure!

If your doctor thinks conventional medicine is a cancer patient's best bet, he should read this story from one of our members...

"I was the worst case of leukemia the Mayo Clinic had seen in 20 years," Ralph Snyder wrote us. "My whole immune system had shut down. My left leg turned black. I went through chemotherapy and whatever else they gave me, but nothing worked very well. My blood counts were very bad and I went home weighing 80 pounds less."

"I needed a miracle...

"And that's when one really happened...A booklet arrived in the mail from Health Sciences Institute. As soon as I took the treatment HSI told me about, my blood counts started improving! I got better and better. Gained back the 80 pounds I lost and then some. I felt great.

"My oncologist at the Mayo Clinic could hardly believe what he saw.

"Right then and there they started calling me THE MIRACLE MAN. It was five years ago and I'm still cancer-free."

Congratulations, Ralph! We share your joy.

The secret is mother's milk

The natural food that saved Ralph Snyder's life is lactoferrin. It's found in the breast milk that mothers feed newborn babies (and colts and calves—the compound is found in most mammals' milk).

This remarkable substance in "first milk" provides powerful immune chemicals to the newborn. And you can get it *only* from Mother Nature. Makers of synthetic formula have tried—and failed—for years to copy the disease-fighting properties of breast milk.

Lactoferrin was one of the first natural cancer therapies we ever reported, *years* ahead of other alternative health experts.

But now it's *just one of six powerful, safe anti-cancer supplements* you'll discover in our free Special Research Alert on how to fight cancer and win. The alert is called *6 Natural Cancer Cures THEY DON'T WANT YOU TO HAVE.* We send a copy to everyone who joins HSI.

Up to 95 percent chance of *preventing* cancer

Ralph Snyder is living testimony that lactoferrin really does work, as do the other proven cancer therapies in *6 Natural Cancer Cures THEY DON'T WANT YOU TO HAVE.* And like the two I mentioned earlier in this little book, lactoferrin is a food supplement that can benefit you now even if you're completely healthy.

It's entirely possible the supplements in this free

Special Research Alert can save you from ever getting cancer in the first place.

You see, alternative cancer experts the world over focus on *building* the immune system, not destroying it the way conventional treatments do. Many of the supplements in your free report not only battle cancer but also fight viruses, bacteria and fungal infections as well.

Conventional medicine's tragic ignorance

The ignorance of America's medical establishment is *known* to hurt children with cancer whose lives could be saved by immune-supporting supplements.

For some reason, children respond better to chemotherapy than adults do, but the little ones often fall prey to infections because the toxic treatment ravages their immune systems.

But the shameless abuses of conventional medicine get even worse...

Whistleblower refused to remain silent about drug company conspiracy

One of the cancer remedies in your free report is a plant extract <u>10,000 times stronger than top chemotherapy drugs</u>. And safer, to boot. This is probably the most famous scoop we ever published.

Yet we wouldn't have known a thing about it if not for a courageous insider at a major pharmaceutical company. This man saw that the natural remedy could turn out to be the most life-saving substance on earth. <u>He refused to stand by</u>

and let the drug giant conceal it from the public forever.

Here's the shameless scam...

Big drug companies are well aware of the healing powers of certain plants, but these natural compounds can't be patented. There's no profit in them for the drug giants. *Their game is to try to __copy__ the natural cure—to create a synthetic, patentable form and reap billions.*

The drug company in this case identified a rain-forest tree from the Amazon with explosive cancer-fighting potential. Certain extracts from the plant actually seek out, attack and destroy cancer cells.

Unlike chemotherapy, which kills BOTH cancer cells and healthy ones, the rain-forest remedy can tell the difference. How can that be?

Compounds in this plant are attracted to a specific enzyme found in the cell walls of cancer tumors. So the plant remedy can hone in on cancer like a laser-guided missile—without damaging your healthy cells. In other words, this is...

One of the most important medical discoveries in history

But did the big drug company call a news conference? Rush out a news release? Publish their findings in a major medical journal?

The answers are: No, no, and no. They kept the whole thing a secret for seven years while they tried to concoct a synthetic version that had the same healing powers.

And when they failed to come up with something they could patent, their plan was to bury the natural discovery and never tell a soul...while around the world, millions would suffer and die needlessly.

Thank God, someone with a conscience kept that from happening, and the news broke first in our Health Sciences Institute monthly alert.

If you or someone you love is struggling against cancer, you couldn't begin to put a dollar value on the information in our Special Report, *6 Natural Cancer Cures THEY DON'T WANT YOU TO HAVE*. But we're not asking a dime for it. The report is our free gift to you just for taking a trial membership in Health Sciences Institute.

There's no obligation, if for any reason you're not fully satisfied, you can have all your money back and keep the report. Join today by sending your Membership Application

Chapter Thirteen

Osteoporosis "experts" are wrong about calcium

Too much calcium could be destroying your health

The real problem is calcium *loss*, not lack of calcium intake. And a natural cure cuts calcium loss by more than two-thirds!

Calcium supplements are <u>not</u> the solution to osteoporosis. *In fact, you're probably overloaded with calcium and it's making you sicker.* The "experts" got it all wrong—again.

And by the way, I'm talking to men as well as women. Bone loss is a major cause of disability, hip fractures and death for *everybody over 50*. This is an epidemic.

In a first-ever report on bone health, the U.S. Surgeon General said <u>half of all older Americans</u> will be in danger of low bone density and osteoporosis.

More bogus solutions designed to line corporate pockets

Where most of us see a crisis, the pharmaceutical industry sees a gold mine. From their viewpoint, what could be better? Seniors are the fastest growing age group, half of them suffer bone loss, and the disease takes decades to kill them.

The way the drug giants see it, we're suckers who will be buying pills for years! Flip on the TV and you'll see tons of ads for prescription drugs to build bone mass.

These ads remind me of those cheery, feel-good ads for Vioxx. You know, the ads that vanished overnight when the joint-pain drug was pulled off the market for making people's hearts stop.

But bone loss is a case where the most popular supplement has problems, too. I'm talking about calcium, which millions of people are popping in doses of up to a gram a day (1000 milligrams)—or even more. The truth is...

You may need only about a tenth of the calcium that U.S. health authorities recommend

Did you know much of this calcium never gets anywhere near your bones? It piles up in your soft tissues where it can actually harm you.

<u>In fact, the excess calcium buries itself in your artery walls and muscle cells where it contributes to high blood pressure and hardening of the arteries</u>.

Why do you think doctors give you calcium channel blockers for high blood pressure?

Good grief, what's going on here? We're drinking milk and stuffing ourselves with calcium supplements, it's not working and our bones are still wasting away, and we're on prescription drugs for high blood pressure?

Stop! Let Health Sciences Institute sort it out!

Our expert contributors got on the case and found you

can save your bones with just 125 milligrams of calcium a day—about a tenth of the typical dose. You just need to make sure the calcium goes where you need it and not to your soft tissues.

How do you do that? Once again, nature has the answer—and we published it as another first for Health Sciences Institute.

Researchers studied the humble oyster to learn how it takes up available calcium and makes it into a hard outer shell. It turns out the secret is *biologically active proteins and enzymes*.

It's thought that these bioactive ingredients from the oyster shell actually pull calcium out of the body's soft tissues, where it can cause damage, and redirect it to the bones to hopefully make them stronger.

And here's the good news: scientists found a way to extract the oyster's secret and create a safe, effective supplement.

Three herbs from Asia seal the deal

To render the formula even more potent, the researchers included three Asian herbs known to <u>inhibit bone loss, heal bone injuries, and prevent degeneration of bone and cartilage</u>.

<u>The first studies show the supplement increased bone density by a staggering 27 percent</u>!

And at the same time, <u>it slashed loss of calcium by 69 percent</u>—more than two-thirds! So the supplement (1) builds your bones, (2) uses only 125 milligrams of calcium to do it, (3) cuts your calcium loss to a fraction of what it was, and (4) spares your arteries—all at the same time.

Receive this health secret and dozens more

When you become a member of Health Sciences

You can look better, too!

In Japan, the nicest compliment you can pay a woman is to say she's looking toki. The word means "skin of a porcelain doll." And *Toki* is the trade name of a second supplement we describe in the free Special Research Alert.

This is another Health Sciences Institute first, and you don't want to miss it.

You'll read about how this Japanese discovery wipes out wrinkles, moisturizes your skin AND reduces joint pain—all in one package.

In one study, four out of five women reported an improved complexion, and 70 percent of them reported relief from joint pain, too. (Sounds weird, but you'll discover why it works this way in the free report).

Send for yours now!

Cut Calcium Loss By 69%

**One of 8
Special Research Alerts
for New Members**

Institute, you'll receive all the details in a Special Research Alert, *Cut Calcium Loss By 69%*. New members receive a total of 8 free Alerts—on cancer, heart disease, diabetes, Alzheimer's, energy, incontinence, and prostate health—in addition to the bone health report.

Just fill out the membership application I sent with this book using the postage-paid envelope.

Chapter Fourteen

Get rid of your allergies for good!

A lifetime on pills? No way!

One patient reports her symptoms are gone forever <u>after one bottle</u>...

The major drug companies aren't looking for an allergy cure. They don't even think about it.

Their products treat only *symptoms.* Anti-inflammatories for the headaches and muscle pain. Decongestants to clear up your sinuses and nasal passages. Inhalers so you can breathe. Antihistamines for everything.

But all of these drugs have side effects. Some can raise your blood pressure, others can make you sleepy, and still others may keep you awake all night. But those are nothing when you consider the *serious* side effects.

For instance, some can destroy your liver. And many labels carry a warning for men with prostate problems. Meaning most men over 50 should think twice before taking these pills.

Almost a decade ago, the most popular prescription allergy medicine at the time, Seldane, was pulled off the market because it turned out to be extremely dangerous.

Nowhere else to go

In spite of the dangers, most allergy victims shrug and take the pills anyway. Many people take the drugs all the time—24 hours a day, seven days a week, 365 days a year. It's scary.

What can you do? You can't afford to be sick all the time.

It's a drug manufacturer's dream! It's a money machine!

At Health Sciences Institute, we look at things differently. We don't want you to keep coming back for more. We want you to get well for good.

What's more, we think there's a natural solution for every health problem...somewhere...if you look hard enough. And we don't mean just a way to stifle the symptoms. We mean something that gets to the *root cause* of the problem.

Another Health Sciences Institute "first"

We combed the globe for years and pumped our network of alternative health professionals and scientists. And finally, our research turned up an astounding herbal formula that can bring you fast, safe relief without drugs.

But it's better than that. *Many people who have tried it say that after the first bottle they don't need to take any more*. Their allergy symptoms go away <u>for good</u>. Just listen to a real-life case...

Rose's allergy-induced asthma was serious. She had to go to the emergency room so often she was practically on a first-name basis with the employees.

She'd suffered from the disease for a large part of her life. She used three different inhalers up to four times a day, as well as using Flonase for about 15 years. And if the

94

asthma didn't kill her, the cost of all the drugs and other treatments came close!

Finally, Rose decided to stop the Flonase. Like a lot of people, she just wanted to feel better without the side effects. But shortly after she quit the drug she was exposed to cats, one of her major allergens, and ended up back in the ER again.

Lifelong problem solved in four days

Then Rose heard about the new herbal therapy. She tried it, and something truly amazing happened. In only four days she was feeling so good, she decided to put the cure to the test. She went to visit a friend with cats.

A life-threatening risk? Not this time! Rose had no problem. What's more, she drank alcohol, ate dairy and even snacked on nuts—actions that might have sent her to the ER only days before. And you know what?

For the first time in decades, Rose didn't have an attack...

And she didn't use her inhalers once!

Rose's experiment falls under the "Do Not Try This at Home" category. You should consult a health professional first about ANY matter that affects your health and well-being.

But her story is remarkable, and it's just one of many. Not only does this breakthrough remedy work for most people, it works fast.

HSI Advisory Panel Member, Dr. Cass, was one of the first clinicians to evaluate the new breakthrough. She told us, "Even in cases where a patient's allergic symptoms were severe and unresponsive to traditional and alternative therapies, the formula brought about almost immediate and profound relief within 30-40 minutes."

Formula's owner turned down $15 million for the rights

We learned about the new breakthrough from a member of our network—in this case, an investor who's always on the lookout for natural cures. He was so impressed with the new herbal formula, he offered the doctor who invented it $10 million for exclusive rights.

And when the doctor turned him down, the investor upped the offer to $15 million!

The investor was so impressed because he'd seen it clear up a child's severe allergy attack in his own home in thirty minutes. He was shocked at how quickly the boy recovered. What's more, he could *see* the difference: The boy's face went from red and swollen to totally normal, right before his eyes.

Our investor friend managed to get the distribution rights and helped the doctor create a brand-spanking-new manufacturing facility (price-tag: $6 million). There the doctor and his family prepare the ten-herb formula to the most *exacting standards*—and in *total secrecy*, to keep anyone from stealing this non-patentable natural formula.

The herbs in the formula may be found in other allergy remedies, but in this case the herbs are fermented enzymatically. As each herb ferments, the manufacturing team captures the volatile oils and aromatics that would escape into the air otherwise. Then, later in the process, they put them back into the product.

We'll rush you a FREE Special Research Alert with all the details on the new allergy formula as soon as you become a member of Health Sciences Institute.

You'll find your Membership Application in this envelope.

Chapter Fifteen

Melt away migraines
in 6.5 minutes!

Four weeds from the side of the road outperform any painkiller you can buy

Here at HSI we receive all kinds of free samples from alternative medicine researchers all over the world. Most of these remedies don't meet our standards, so our readers never hear about them.

But the migraine solution in this chapter passed every test. It brings TOTAL RELIEF to so many people who try it. It works FAST. It's totally SAFE. It's INEXPENSIVE and it's EASY TO GET.

30-year problem solved in seconds

One of our HSI colleagues has been fighting migraines for 30 years. She's tried everything from powerful prescription painkillers to injections to nasal sprays. She told us her headache pain was so intense, she was willing to try anything.

So whenever we'd receive a promising migraine remedy, our friend got first dibs on the free sample. One day, we received a bottle of a sublingual (under-the-tongue) spray, and as usual we passed it on to her.

The next time she developed a migraine she pulled it out. A couple of quick spritzes and...

She could feel the pain dulling instantly

What's more, she didn't feel any negative side effects—no "rebound" headache, no nasty taste, and no upset stomach.

Of course, we wanted more evidence—and we found it. A double-blind, placebo-controlled study done by the makers of this product confirms what our colleague told us. Of those test subjects who tried the spray, <u>two out of three reported full to complete improvement</u>. But here's what's really amazing...

They got relief in just six and a half minutes, on average!

There's more: a lot of the people who didn't get TOTAL relief reported SOME relief. The overall success rate for this natural remedy was just about nine out of ten.

What's in it? Just weeds you could pick from the side of the road! It's a homeopathic blend of four traditional herbs: feverfew, goldenseal, dandelion and polyporus officinalis.

The lead ingredient, feverfew, is a traditional herb for migraines. We can show you a whole folder full of clinical studies that prove it works.

The other three ingredients aren't usually called migraine remedies. But when you look at their track records, it's easy to see why they work with feverfew to produce the fast relief so many patients report. You've probably heard of goldenseal as a cold and flu therapy, but it's also a sedative and an anti-inflammatory.

But perhaps the biggest breakthrough here is the concept of taking the painkiller under your tongue. That bypasses your digestive system and rushes the medicine right to your brain.

We'll tell you where to find this four-herb spray in a Special Report called ***Pain Free for Life***—our gift to you when you become a member of HSI. The report also has some tips and cautions to make sure you get the maximum benefit (for instance, you may not want to take certain prescription and OTC drugs at the same time).

To receive ***Pain Free for Life***, send in the Membership Application enclosed with this book in the postage-paid envelope today. There are extra applications at the end of the book, you can pass on to friends.

And just in case they find a way to make dandelion illegal and yank the spray off the market...

We don't want you to be without an answer to migraine pain, so here's another natural solution you can get any time.

Scientists at the University of Munich proved it works in a study of extreme migraine sufferers. These people were really hard cases. If you wanted to take part in the study, the researchers accepted you only if you suffered at least three migraines a month for the preceding year. Ouch!

The double-blind, placebo-controlled test showed this herb *slashed the number of headaches by well over half.*

And when the folks in the test DID get a headache, they told their doctors the episode was shorter and the pain was less.

In other words, dear FDA, this is for real

The herb I'm talking about is butterbur. Yes, another "useless weed" found on the banks of streams and rivers in most of the world—in Europe, Asia and North America. Our ancestors prized its medicinal qualities for thousands of years. They even tried it against the Black Death 650 years ago (it didn't work, I have to admit).

But the butterbur that gave such amazing relief in the Munich study is something new. It's a potent extract that reduced the number of headaches per month *by more than half.*

When I say it's new, I mean it's new to Americans. Europeans have used the extract safely for 30 years.

Join us as a member of Health Sciences Institute and get our free report, *Pain Free for Life*. You'll get all the details on the butterbur extract AND the powerful sublingual spray that eliminates most headaches in minutes.

Butterbur from your doctor? Fat chance!

Is it likely your doctor would ever tell you about butterbur...or about the sublingual migraine spray...or about the heart and cancer remedies and all the other solutions in this little book?

I don't think so.

Don't get me wrong. Conventional medicine has its place. If there's a smallpox epidemic or I'm in a car accident or I need to have my appendix removed, I'll head straight for a regular hospital.

They can fix me up. If the doctors don't believe in butterbur or Echinacea, we'll talk about it later.

But that leaves a whole range of health conditions where natural medicine has better answers. Powerful multibillion interests have kept these natural answers out of our medical schools, out of our medical journals and out of our country.

It's not our personal doctors who keep these treatments away from us. They don't even know about them. And the drug industry spends billions of dollars to make sure they don't.

But you CAN learn about these health solutions.

Here's how to get started...

Chapter Sixteen

Your Membership Privileges

8 Free Special Alerts...and much more

When you join Health Sciences Institute, you receive the 8 FREE Special Research Alerts I've described in these pages. In fact, you can get four more—a total of 12 reports—by taking a two-year membership.

But valuable as they are, the free Special Research Alerts are just the beginning of your membership privileges when you join Health Sciences Institute.

In fact, all the cures in the Research Alerts appeared *first* in one of our monthly bulletins.

As a member, you receive a new, fresh 8-page report every month with breaking news on the very latest developments in the world of alternative health. Every breakthrough in this book appeared first in the monthly newsletter.

If you've never seen this publication before, you're in for a surprise...

We don't report the news—we make the news

With our home office staff, plus the 19 renowned doctors and researchers on our Advisory Panel, PLUS our network of informants in universities, clinics, institutes and laboratories all over the world...

We bring you original discoveries and path-breaking research never before published. These are stories you will see nowhere else. Nearly every treatment I've described in this book was a Health Sciences Institute scoop.

You'll find out what I mean—one issue of our monthly alert will make you a believer. But membership goes beyond that...

You can receive an informative e-mail each and every day

That's right. You get more than a monthly issue. Every day, we send an e-mail Alert with new discoveries as well as our comments on the day's health news.

The e-mail Alerts briefed our members on the Vioxx fiasco three years before the drug was pulled off the shelves. And we tell you the truth about those ridiculous studies that "prove" natural remedies such as vitamin C or E or Echinacea don't work. It seems like every day there's another one.

They're mostly nonsense designed to mislead you.

This is important, because the medical establishment works around the clock to attack natural medicine. The daily e-Alert provides a valuable balance to their daily, non-stop disinformation campaign.

Unlimited access to our priceless database of health information

There's no price I could possibly put on this next benefit: You can search our Internet archives for whatever we've published on any <u>health subject you want</u>.

It's a <u>complete health library</u>—a virtual alternative health encyclopedia, at your fingertips. And our search engine finds what you want *fast*.

That means if there's something you need to know now, you can pull up everything we've published about it within seconds. Our huge archive includes not only our 8-page monthly issues but also thousands of daily e-mail Alerts. They're all a mouse-click away in the online archive.

"We are family" —a big, caring family

As a member of Health Sciences Institute, you also get free admission to the HSI Internet Forums. You've joined a family, a warm, supportive group of people who are ready to share their lifesaving, health-savvy insights and experiences with you whenever you're in need.

Want to know how one of our recommendations works before *you* try it? No problem! Ask our other members. They'll tell you, and you'll see our solutions really do work.

In fact, link up with our 90,000-strong members and ask them any question you want. No matter what your medical problem, I guarantee you that other members have "been there, done that" and they can tell you what worked for them.

A quality filter to protect you

Sad to say, there are no formal quality standards for supplements and alternative remedies. Alternative medicine can be like the Wild West. But you have our assurance that we carefully screen suppliers and products and publish information about ONLY THE BEST.

By the way, that may not mean the biggest or most famous. We've found that lesser-known firms often offer the highest quality.

Discounts and priority treatment, too

If you've read this book, you know that some of the remedies and supplements we discuss aren't easy to find. Some are rare, and many have only one source. Often, there's only one source that WE trust.

As a result, supplies can be tight, and when that happens we intervene on behalf of our members. You're not just the first to *know* about new remedies, you're the first to get them. Your membership puts you at the front of the line.

What's more, in many cases we're able to negotiate special deals and discounts for our members—for one thing, the folks on our Advisory Panel are often on the research teams that develop the treatments.

Get in on the ground floor of new research

From time to time we're able to offer members the chance to take part in research trials on the most promising new breakthroughs. That means you might receive the treatment at greatly reduced cost or even FREE.

What's more, if you have an "incurable" health condition and nowhere else to turn, this means you don't have to wait years for a new discovery that could bring you healing and relief. We believe you have the right to make your own decisions.

Every New Member Receives 8 Free Reports

You'll never again put up with a medical problem for years...

Or even lose someone you love...

Only to discover there was a cure all along, but America's health police kept it from you!

Health Sciences Institute is your vital, life-saving information pipeline to the outside world—a world of cures the billion-dollar drug giants don't want us to know.

FREE REPORT #1:
6 Natural Cancer Cures
THEY DON'T WANT YOU TO HAVE

The rain-forest plant that's 10,000 times stronger than top chemotherapy drugs—and kills ONLY cancer cells. A big drug company tried to conceal it forever...The marvelous mushroom extract that eliminated ALL cancer cells in more than half the people tested...A wheat germ compound discovered by the same Nobel Prize winner who discovered vitamin C. It reduces cancer fatalities by an incredible 62 percent!...**PLUS THREE OTHER NATURAL CANCER-FIGHTERS**—and you can take five of them to prevent cancer, too.

FREE REPORT #2:
Diabetes Defeated: From Insulin-Dependent to Non-Diabetic in 6 Weeks Flat

Health Sciences Institute Panelist Jon Barron helped develop a revolutionary five-herb formula that could mean salvation for millions. *82 percent who try it get better,* and the product is so popular the maker can barely keep it in stock! Blood sugar levels plunge 20 percent, 29 percent, 35 percent, 51 percent— *within weeks.* But it gets even better: Cholesterol tumbles, too!

FREE REPORT #3:
Natural Energy Boosters

Count us in! The secret is a rare type of sugar not found in any food. Your body has to make its own, in a complex process that just plain doesn't work in people who suffer fatigue. Now this vital nutrient is available for the first time as a supplement, and it has people running sprints who used to be too tired to climb a flight of stairs! The rare sugar (harmless to diabetics) is a critical building block for ATP—the vital enzyme you need to energize each and every one of your cells.

FREE REPORT #4:
Stop Memory Loss Dead in its Tracks

One herb *stops the progress* of Alzheimer's and another actually *reverses* it. You'll learn both in this free Special

Research Alert. A respected scientist says the nutrients "may reverse approximately 12 years of decline" —and that goes for ALL of us who have memory problems. *Seven out of ten experience <u>measurable</u> memory improvement within four weeks.*

FREE REPORT #5:
Cut Calcium Loss By 69%: Today's Medicines for Women

The osteoporosis "experts" are wrong about calcium. Over-supplementing with calcium may be bad for your health because most of it ends up in your soft tissues, where it causes harm. The real problem is calcium *loss,* not a deficiency of calcium in your diet. And this Special Research Alert features a natural cure that cuts calcium loss *by more than two-thirds.* Another Health Sciences Institute first, and the early results are astounding!

FREE REPORT #6:
The Secret Cures for Heart Disease

Cuts cholesterol sharply in 30 days...Reduces the number of angina episodes *by half, without side effects* (much better than the leading prescription drug)...Brings down blood pressure...And you may even lose a few pounds without dieting! In a placebo-controlled study, patients with final-stage congestive heart failure got better in *two weeks.* **It may sound like five different herbs, but in fact, it's just one!** Sometimes we find a natural remedy that does so many things, it's hard even for us to believe it. But this is for real. PLUS: The heart-failure remedy we'd want with us on a desert island. Results are just starting to come in, but it may be the most promising natural heart and stroke solution ever found. Another HSI first.

FREE REPORT #7:
The Powerful Prostate Antidote: Today's Medicines for Men

Traditional Vietnamese medicine is one of the most overlooked treasures in the world—but not by us! This report brings you a rare prostate herb so effective, Vietnamese authorities don't want it to leave the country. Solves nine out of ten enlarged prostate problems and totally eliminates prostate tumors. We've found an American source for you.

FREE REPORT #8:
Control Your Bladder the Natural Way

Who wants to wear Depends or plan their life around bathroom breaks? Nobody, that's who. Now you don't have to. HSI Panelist Allan Spreen, M.D., was one of the brains behind bringing this natural solution for bladder support. After reviewing every food or nutrient in the world that's believed to support bladder health, this team created a formula that puts you back in charge.

Sign up for a Two-Year Membership and Get 4 More Free Reports!

FREE REPORT #9:
Pain Free for Life

When international scientists decided to cure arthritis, they first looked at native peoples who never get the disease—and analyzed what they ate. After two decades of research, the surprising result is the extract of a New Zealand mussel. It's related to the omega-3 fatty acids that help prevent heart disease, and it beats the pants off drug-company anti-inflammatories—with NO side effects. *ALSO IN THIS REPORT: A sublingual (under-the-tongue) herbal spray that relieves migraines in two out of three patients—in minutes.* **PLUS: Six more natural painkillers.**

FREE REPORT #10:
Get Rid of Your Allergies for Good

Many people who try this herbal remedy say they don't need to take any more after the first bottle. *Their allergy symptoms go away for good.* Most of us would settle for a lot less than that! It's no surprise one of America's leading supplement manufacturers offered $15 million for the rights, and the developer turned him down. This Special Research Alert explains what it is, how it works, and where to get it.

FREE REPORT #11:
Clear Up The Flu In 8 Hours Flat

Back in the dark days of the Cold War, the Russian military needed to find an antidote to the very germ warfare agents they planned to use on us! Their microbiologists set out to analyze 600 products that <u>protect against powerful killers like anthrax</u>. In the pages of this Special Research Alert, you'll learn the very best they found: a totally safe natural remedy that wipes out cold and flu with amazing speed. I'm not talking about symptomatic relief. I'm talking about a total cure.

And there's a strange angle here. We don't know why, but a major TV network planned to air a prime-time special about this super-germ-killer, and then abruptly cancelled it. Pressure from big advertisers? You be the judge. But at a time of terrorism AND new super-viruses such as SARS and avian flu, no home should be without this remedy.

FREE REPORT #12:
Fat-Burning Aids from the Underground

This is the report the diet industry does NOT want you to read. They profit most when you know the least. In the pages of this Special Research Alert, you'll discover **the fatless fat** that tastes like butter but won't add weight...**a fat-gobbling body chemical that exists in your blood right now**. Here's how to wake it up with simple, little-known tricks!...**PLUS: Nature's most surprising fat**

fighter blocks fat absorption, keeps your appetite in check and keeps your energy high. Absolutely the simplest and best way to lose weight. You feel full and satisfied all the time, safely.

FAST REPLY BONUS!

Join right away and as a way to thank you for your membership, we'll also send you...

Vital Health Secrets

- *Don't even think about cataract surgery till you've read this.* Studies show natural eye drops treat up to 100 percent of patients without drugs or surgery. A few drops a day and cataracts go away. **PLUS: Our best solution for macular degeneration**.

- **Turn stress or depression to happiness in four days.** This anti-aging secret of the rich and powerful (not a hormone) is now available to all for the first time, as a supplement. Truly incredible.

AND THERE'S MORE: Our best solution to **periodontal disease**. It's so easy you'll kick yourself—or the boneheaded FDA people who discouraged it...An herbal tea extract that **lowers blood sugar** and supports weight loss...A grape extract (not *that* one, something new!) that improves or totally **cures psoriasis** for eight out of ten.

You receive all eight solutions in **Vital Health Secrets** as our thanks for replying fast.

All this knowledge and more for pennies a day!

If you accept this special invitation now, you can gain unbridled access to all this information—everything I've described—for about a penny-and-a-half a day.

Surely your health is worth more than that. And surely it's worth more than that to support our efforts to publish the truth about big drug companies and the breakthrough treatments they try to keep from us.

You take no risk

Naturally, you're under no obligation to remain a member if you're not satisfied. Look over the 8 FREE Special Research Alerts (12 for two-year members). Read one or two monthly issues. Surf our extensive online archives—ask our search engine any health question you like. Then...

If you're unhappy AT ANY TIME, FOR ANY REASON, just let us know and we'll send you a prompt refund for all remaining issues on your subscription. You keep the free reports and anything else we've sent you, with our compliments.

I enclosed a loose reply form and postage-paid envelope with this little book. But if you misplaced them, no problem. You'll find extra application forms in the back of this book.

We'd love to have you!

For your health and freedom,

Dr. Benjamin Ross

Health Sciences Institute
No-Risk Introductory Membership Application

☐ **YES!** Rush me 8 FREE Special Research Alerts and enter my one-year (12-issue) introductory membership to Health Sciences Institute for $49 ($25 off reg. rate). (See reverse for more about the free gifts). I understand I may cancel at any time, receive a full refund on all remaining issues, and the free gifts are mine to keep. (021)

☐ **BEST DEAL:** I prefer a two-year membership for $79 because that way I receive 4 MORE FREE GIFTS for a total of 12, AND I save $69 off the regular rate. The same refund guarantee applies.(022)

PAYMENT OPTIONS:

☐ My payment is enclosed for $49 ($79 for two years).
Make checks payable to Health Sciences Institute.
(Maryland residents please add 5% sales tax.)

☐ Charge my credit card: ☐ VISA ☐ MC ☐ AMEX ☐ Discover

Card Number   Exp. Date

Name

Signature

Address

City/State/Zip Code

Phone Number *(In case we have a question about your order.)*

E-mail *(If you wish to receive our FREE e-Alert service. We do not release your e-mail address to third parties.)*

Mail to: Health Sciences Institute, Order Processing Center
P.O. Box 925, Frederick, MD 21705-9913

CIR-P

D600DOM

All New Members Receive
8 FREE GIFTS

6 Natural Cancer Cures THEY DON'T WANT YOU

Cut Calcium Loss By 69%: Today's Medicines for Women

HSI

Diabetes Defeated: From Insulin Dependent to Non-Diabetic in 6

The Secret Cures for Heart Disease

HSI

Natural Energy Booster

The Powerful Prostate Antidote: Today's Medicine's for Men

HSI

Stop Memory Loss Dead in its

Control Your Bladder the Natural Way

HSI

Join for two years and receive
4 MORE FREE GIFTS

Pain Free for Life

HSI

Clear up the Flu IN 8 HOURS FLAT

HSI

Get Rid of Your Allergies for Good

HSI

FAT-BURNING AIDS FROM THE UNDERGROUND

HSI

REPLY FAST AND
GET A BONUS GIFT!

Apply for membership within two weeks and you also receive:

Vital Health Secrets

HSI

YOU TAKE NO RISK WHEN YOU JOIN

If for any reason you're not delighted with your Membership benefits, just drop us a note to cancel AT ANY TIME. We'll send you a prompt and courteous refund on all unmailed issues. The free gifts and any issues you've received are yours to keep. And thanks for trying us!

Health Sciences Institute
No-Risk Introductory Membership Application

☐ **YES!** Rush me 8 FREE Special Research Alerts and enter my one-year (12-issue) introductory membership to Health Sciences Institute for $49 ($25 off reg. rate). (See reverse for more about the free gifts). I understand I may cancel at any time, receive a full refund on all remaining issues, and the free gifts are mine to keep. (021)

☐ **BEST DEAL:** I prefer a two-year membership for $79 because that way I receive 4 MORE FREE GIFTS for a total of 12, AND I save $69 off the regular rate. The same refund guarantee applies.(022)

PAYMENT OPTIONS:

☐ My payment is enclosed for $49 ($79 for two years). Make checks payable to Health Sciences Institute.
   (Maryland residents please add 5% sales tax.)

☐ Charge my credit card: ☐ VISA ☐ MC ☐ AMEX ☐ Discover

Card Number _____ Exp. Date _____

Name _____

Signature _____

Address _____

City/State/Zip Code _____

Phone Number *(In case we have a question about your order.)* _____

E-mail *(If you wish to receive our FREE e-Alert service. We do not release your e-mail address to third parties.)* _____

Mail to: Health Sciences Institute, Order Processing Center
P.O. Box 925, Frederick, MD 21705-9913

D600DOM

All New Members Receive
8 FREE GIFTS

6 Natural Cancer Cures THEY DON'T WANT YOU

Cut Calcium Loss By 69%: Today's Medicines for Women

HSI

Diabetes Defeated: From Insulin Dependent to Non-Diabetic in 6

The Secret Cures for Heart Disease

HSI

Natural Energy Booster

The Powerful Prostate Antidote: Today's Medicine's for Men

HSI

Stop Memory Loss Dead in its

Control Your Bladder the Natural Way

HSI

Join for two years and receive
4 MORE FREE GIFTS

Pain Free for Life

HSI

Clear up the Flu IN 8 HOURS FLAT

HSI

Get Rid of Your Allergies for Good

HSI

FAT-BURNING AIDS FROM THE UNDERGROUND

HSI

REPLY FAST AND
GET A BONUS GIFT!

Apply for membership within two weeks and you also receive:

Vital Health Secrets

HSI

YOU TAKE NO RISK WHEN YOU JOIN

If for any reason you're not delighted with your Membership benefits, just drop us a note to cancel AT ANY TIME. We'll send you a prompt and courteous refund on all unmailed issues. The free gifts and any issues you've received are yours to keep. And thanks for trying us!

All New Members Receive
8 FREE GIFTS

6 Natural Cancer Cures THEY DON'T WANT YOU

Cut Calcium Loss By 69%: Today's Medicines for Women

HSI

Diabetes Defeated: From Insulin Dependent to Non-Diabetic in 5

The Secret Cures for Heart Disease

HSI

Natural Energy Booster

The Powerful Prostate Antidote: Today's Medicine's for Men

HSI

Stop Memory Loss Dead in its

Control Your Bladder the Natural Way

HSI

Join for two years and receive
4 MORE FREE GIFTS

Pain Free for Life

HSI

Clear up the Flu IN 8 HOURS FLAT

HSI

Get Rid of Your Allergies for Good

HSI

FAT-BURNING AIDS FROM THE UNDERGROUND

HSI

REPLY FAST AND
GET A BONUS GIFT!

Apply for membership within two weeks and you also receive:

Vital Health Secrets

HSI

YOU TAKE NO RISK WHEN YOU JOIN

If for any reason you're not delighted with your Membership benefits, just drop us a note to cancel AT ANY TIME. We'll send you a prompt and courteous refund on all unmailed issues. The free gifts and any issues you've received are yours to keep. And thanks for trying us!

Health Sciences Institute
No-Risk Introductory Membership Application

❏ **YES!** Rush me 8 FREE Special Research Alerts and enter my one-year (12-issue) introductory membership to Health Sciences Institute for $49 ($25 off reg. rate). (See reverse for more about the free gifts). I understand I may cancel at any time, receive a full refund on all remaining issues, and the free gifts are mine to keep. (021)

❏ **BEST DEAL:** I prefer a two-year membership for $79 because that way I receive 4 MORE FREE GIFTS for a total of 12, AND I save $69 off the regular rate. The same refund guarantee applies.(022)

PAYMENT OPTIONS:

❏ My payment is enclosed for $49 ($79 for two years).
Make checks payable to Health Sciences Institute.
(Maryland residents please add 5% sales tax.)

❏ Charge my credit card: ❏ VISA ❏ MC ❏ AMEX ❏ Discover

Card Number   Exp. Date

Name

Signature

Address

City/State/Zip Code

Phone Number *(In case we have a question about your order.)*

E-mail *(If you wish to receive our FREE e-Alert service. We do not release your e-mail address to third parties.)*

**Mail to: Health Sciences Institute, Order Processing Center
P.O. Box 925, Frederick, MD 21705-9913**

CIR-P

D600DOM

DHS1007-RPLY

T1/12 T2/24

All New Members Receive
8 FREE GIFTS

6 Natural Cancer Cures THEY DON'T WANT YOU

Diabetes Defeated: From Insulin Dependent to Non-Diabetic in 6

Natural Energy Booster

Stop Memory Loss Dead in its

Cut Calcium Loss By 69%: Today's Medicines for Women

HSI

The Secret Cures for Heart Disease

HSI

The Powerful Prostate Antidote: Today's Medicine's for Men

HSI

Control Your Bladder the Natural Way

HSI

Join for two years and receive
4 MORE FREE GIFTS

Pain Free for Life

HSI

Clear up the Flu IN 8 HOURS FLAT

HSI

Get Rid of Your Allergies for Good

HSI

FAT-BURNING AIDS FROM THE UNDERGROUND

HSI

REPLY FAST AND
GET A BONUS GIFT!
Apply for membership within two weeks and you also receive:

Vital Health Secrets

HSI

YOU TAKE NO RISK WHEN YOU JOIN
If for any reason you're not delighted with your Membership benefits, just drop us a note to cancel AT ANY TIME. We'll send you a prompt and courteous refund on all unmailed issues. The free gifts and any issues you've received are yours to keep. And thanks for trying us!